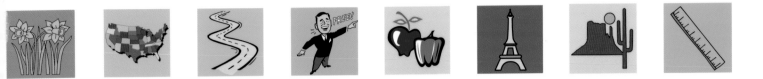

Kristin Einberger & Janelle Sellick

STRENGTHEN
YOUR
MIND

Activities for People
with Early Memory Loss

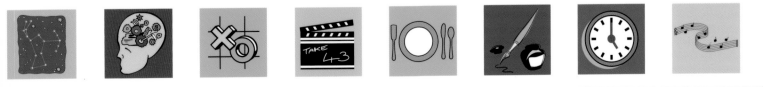

Strengthen Your Mind

Strengthen Your Mind

Activities for People with Early Memory Loss

by

Kristin Einberger

and

Janelle Sellick

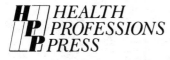
HEALTH PROFESSIONS PRESS

Baltimore • London • Sydney

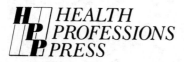

Health Professions Press
Post Office Box 10624
Baltimore, Maryland 21285-0624

www.healthpropress.com

Typeset by Barton Matheson Willse & Worthington, Baltimore, Maryland.
Manufactured in the United States of America by
Versa Press, Inc., East Peoria, Illinois.

Library of Congress Cataloging-in-Publication Data

Einberger, Kristin.
    Strengthen your mind : activities for people with early memory loss / by Kristin Einberger and Janelle Sellick.
       p.   cm.
    ISBN-13: 978-1-932529-31-9 (layflat)
    ISBN-10: 1-932529-31-4 (layflat)
    1. Memory disorders—Exercise therapy.   I. Sellick, Janelle.   II. Title.
    BF376.E36 2007
    616.8'3—dc22   2006029586

British Library Cataloguing in Publication data are available from the British Library.

Contents

Foreword

As a support group leader for families and individuals with Alzheimer's disease for 30 years, I frequently ask about the most difficult manifestations of the disease process. Overwhelmingly, individuals with early memory loss answer, "Not being able to make choices or to plan meaningful use of leisure time." Family care partners' responses mimic those of individuals with early memory loss.

Although several books containing appropriate leisure-time activities have been published in the past, *Strengthen Your Mind: Activities for People with Early Memory Loss* offers a unique presentation of hands-on activity sheets that are both entertaining and therapeutic. These worksheets afford individuals with early memory loss an opportunity to draw on memory that has been stored, yet untapped, for many years and to test recall while simultaneously providing an opportunity for positive interaction with facilitators or family care partners.

I tested two of the A-to-Z Worksheets (*E.T. Phone Home—Famous Movie Lines* and *Red, White, and Blue*) by asking the series of questions to 14 individuals with early memory loss in a support group. It was one of the most exhilarating sessions in years. Everyone participated, including those who usually are the most quiet during the group sessions, and many recalled the experience at the next group meeting.

Chances to feel successful are slim, if not nonexistent, for this overlooked group of adults; *Strengthen Your Mind* reverses the powerful emotion of ongoing failure and replaces it with feelings of joy at succeeding when a reasonable response is positively recorded. In no way do these worksheets seem like a test but instead a fun opportunity to call on stored information. Answering a question correctly validates the individual's feeling of self-worth and underscores that he or she is still a functioning member of his or her personal community.

Accolades to Kristin Einberger and Janelle Sellick for researching and penning this wonderful exploration of remaining memories. Each of the worksheets provides a plethora of information culled from past times. Every family should have a copy of *Strengthen Your Mind,* and all community-based programs (assisted living, adult day health, long-term care, and others) should use this marvelous tome in daily programming.

The authors have found a way to overlook the disease and applaud the humanness of individuals living with Alzheimer's disease.

Joanne Koenig Coste
Author, *Learning to Speak Alzheimer's*

Preface

Over the past several years, the importance of taking part in mentally stimulating activities has become apparent. Healthy older adults, people concerned about their memory, and individuals diagnosed with an early memory loss disorder can all benefit from keeping their minds active. The worksheets within this manual are a wonderful way to begin this "mental exercise"—they help to enhance memory, stimulate the mind, and promote socialization with others.

This book is a product of years of work with people with early memory loss. In 2002, we developed and facilitated one of the first social/educational programs designed specifically for people with early memory loss. As a result, the activities and worksheets in this book have been designed with much input from people with early memory loss and "tested" with early memory loss groups to make sure that they are applicable to the needs and abilities of these individuals. In fact, many of the worksheets have been worked and reworked after suggestions and tips from members of the early memory loss groups. As mentioned in the acknowledgments, we thank these members for their dedication and patience as our idea for this book became a reality.

Today, these worksheets are used as a regular part of these social/educational groups, and they have been a valuable tool for discussion, memory enhancement, and socialization. Whether you are a person concerned about memory, a professional, or a family member of someone with memory loss, we hope you enjoy using these worksheets and that they provide hours of reminiscence, sharing, and mental stimulation.

Acknowledgments

This book is dedicated to the members of Brain Boosters and Mind Boosters, two very special groups in northern California with whom we have had the privilege to work. These wonderful people have served as our inspiration in guiding us through the process of developing activities that were stimulating, educational, and challenging as well as fun. Without them, our thoughts would still be just that. We wish to thank them from the very bottom of our hearts for their perseverance, courage, dedication, humor, and kindness. You are the greatest!

In addition, we would like to thank our immediate families—Mike, Mia, Megan, Derek, and Scott— as well as other members of our families and friends, both for serving as "testing grounds" for the activities and for generating ideas for questions. Dinner-table conversations, vacations, friends' nights out, car trips, long telephone calls—all were so helpful in the development of the book and were deeply appreciated. Many of the suggestions are contained within these activities. Many of the others are being saved for the next book! Our heartfelt thanks also go out to the many professionals with whom we have worked over the last few years, especially to Anne, who spent countless hours listening to our ideas and making suggestions, and to Leah for helping "test" the activities with the Brain Boosters group.

Without the help and caring of all these people, this book would never have come into being.

Introduction

You may have heard about the importance of doing crossword puzzles or playing games to keep your mind active. Although this is certainly good advice, in reality an endless supply of activities can be used to challenge and strengthen your mind. We, the authors, have researched and tested more than 65 topics that we have turned into worksheets that we encourage you to explore. Be prepared to learn about everything, from your five senses, to city nicknames, to chocolate and other desserts.

One of the most important goals of this manual is that you enjoy spending time completing the worksheets. Although getting the correct answers is rewarding, you may find that working with a family member, friend, or neighbor to figure out the answers is even more fun. There are a variety of subjects explored in these worksheets; some questions will be easy for you while others will be more challenging. The worksheets are in a variety of formats, from multiple choice, to fill in the blank, to brainstorming and others. Do not worry if you cannot find the answer to every question on a page; just enjoy taking the time to scout out the answers by talking with others or using reference materials such as the Internet, dictionaries, and encyclopedias to locate your answer. In addition, you may find more than one answer for some questions. Above all, have fun with the manual—the true benefit of the worksheets is participating in the process of finding the answers, not knowing every answer!

Although completing these worksheets is interesting and fun, there are a variety of other benefits that come from using this manual. By participating in mentally challenging activities on a regular basis, you can strengthen and sharpen your mind. The worksheets in this manual will encourage you to research and discuss topics that you may never have had an interest in or even thought of learning about before. With each worksheet that you complete, you will gain a little more knowledge to tuck away and add to a lifetime of learning and experiences. Socializing with others about the worksheets is important also. Completing the worksheets with another person can foster camaraderie and purpose. Simply put, the worksheets contain fun topics of conversation that everyone will enjoy discussing. In addition, interacting with others helps to decrease feelings of loneliness and depression. Finally, the questions on each worksheet can trigger a variety of memories and encourage you to reflect and analyze how things have changed over the decades. As you go about answering the questions on each worksheet, you will find that not only are you enjoying yourself, but you also are stimulating your mind, your senses, and your memory. Enjoy!

INFORMATION FOR FACILITATORS

Not only are the worksheets in this manual beneficial for individuals, but they are also an excellent resource for professionals who work with people who want to strengthen their minds. For these professionals (i.e., *facilitators*), the following are some tips and suggestions to make your sessions as beneficial as they can be.

The answers to each question are listed on the back of each worksheet (i.e., the *answer sheet*). Make sure to look at the bottom of the answer sheet to the *facilitator* section. In this section, you will find valuable tips and suggestions to encourage discussion, find further resources, and expand on the topic. The worksheets are designed to be reproducible. We suggest running enough copies (front side only) for each person whom you are working with. You may even want to provide extra copies for people to take home with them so that they can give them to family members or friends to work together on the topic.

When you gather together to go over the worksheets, make sure that participants are relaxed and focused on the topic before you begin. You can ask them how they liked the worksheet, if they found it easy or difficult, or who they worked with to complete it. When reviewing the questions, encourage people in the group to share their answers. Avoid just "reading off" the answers, and take time to let people share any thoughts, memories, or stories that arise. Make the group feel comfortable by encouraging them to share or by sharing a story of your own. Many of the topics are about common items or cultural icons. Whenever possible, bring in an object (or several) that signifies the topic of the worksheet. For example, one of the worksheets is about foreign currencies. Try to find samples of different currencies that the group can handle. For even more fun, bring in samples of foods such as a variety of chocolates for the *Chocolate, Chocolate, Chocolate* worksheet.

Above all, the most important aspect of the worksheets in this manual is that they spur conversation, encourage sharing, and stimulate the mind. If you have fun with them, then the people you work with will also!

Sensory Activities

Take time to smell the roses. We've all heard this expression over and over, but do we really "hear" it? Do we really heed its advice? Do we use all of our senses to explore our surroundings? All too often, the answer to these questions is *no.* It is our hope as authors of this book that the following activities will help you to do just that—not only to smell the roses but also to savor their beauty using all of your senses.

Everything we know, everything we learn, comes to us from our senses. Let's look at each of our five senses and think about how we can use each one of them to enhance our memories.

HEARING

As we age, most of us experience a decline in our sense of hearing. This makes it imperative that we listen better. We need to minimize distractions around us and really listen to what others are saying. There are many tricks to remembering what we hear, but perhaps the best is to pay attention by listening intently and then repeating what is heard back to yourself, either out loud or silently. Begin to focus on all of the sounds you hear, from the loud honk at the intersection to the faint sound of a leaf falling from a tree. Talk with friends, and listen to music and books on tape.

SMELL

Odors trigger memories more than any of the other five senses. Just think of one of your favorite smells—freshly popped popcorn, your loved one's cologne, freshly mowed grass—and see how many memories come to mind. We can recognize as many as 10,000 smells during our lifetimes. This number decreases as we age, though even at 100 years old we still have the ability to recognize thousands of smells! We need to learn to use this wonderful sense to its fullest potential. Start paying attention to all of the smells you encounter in your everyday life. Take time to smell that rose, that cake in the oven, and that newly laundered shirt.

TASTE

We are born with about 10,000 taste buds. As we grow older, this number decreases. This accounts for the fact that many foods don't taste as strong as they once did. Try eating new foods. There are many delicious ethnic foods now on the market and at restaurants that can provide us with new taste sensations. Add different herbs and spices to those foods that you have always eaten but no longer enjoy as much. Grow some of these herbs yourself. Try new recipes. Pay special attention to the taste of each food you eat, which will help you to store these tastes in your memory.

TOUCH/FEELINGS

Our sense of touch shows us how the world "feels." It informs us of danger, registers what makes us happy or jumpy, and determines whether something feels smooth or rough. Our sense of touch, unlike the other senses, is found all over our bodies. If we are to enhance our memory, it is imperative that we really think about our sense of touch—really pay attention to how things feel and to the feelings we experience as we go through each day. Undertake new projects that require you to touch, such as gardening, cooking, and building things. Play games, and do crossword puzzles. Consider your feelings. Do you feel happy? Mad? Scared? Be aware of the emotions behind your feelings.

VISION

Most of the information we take in about the world is based on what we see. Our sense of vision is the most complex of all of our senses. It allows us countless opportunities for learning and remembering. Learn to "see" with the eyes of a child. Focus on the sight of what you want to remember. Study it. Imagine it. Really see it. Pay attention to all that's around you. Go for walks and "see" everything around you, from the smallest ant to a large truck passing by.

USING ALL OF OUR SENSES

If we isolate each sense and really learn to use it individually, without the help of the other four senses, it will help us to more effectively use our senses all together. The more information we receive through a variety of paths, the more likely we are to remember things. If we truly use all of our senses in combination with one another, we stand the greatest likelihood of being able to enhance our memories.

The activities on the following pages are divided into each of the five senses. The last pages deal with the senses as a whole. On the front of each page is an activity for you to complete. Once you have done this, turn the page. The backside will have answers, ideas, and/or suggestions for completing the activity. There will also be a paragraph at the bottom of the page to give you, a friend, a family member, or a facilitator of your group ideas on how to do more with each activity.

There are countless activities that deal with each of the senses. The ones on the following pages are just the beginning!! Try to engage your different senses as you complete everyday activities; use as many as possible, even if some of them require imagination!! Start truly smelling the roses.

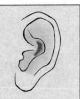

Slogans that Deal with Sound

Each of the following slogans deals with the sense of hearing—with the sound of things. Identify the products that the following slogans advertise, matching them with those on the right. Imagine the sounds as you go.

___ 1. His master's voice

___ 2. It takes a licking and keeps on ticking.

___ 3. Snap, crackle, pop

___ 4. Plop, plop, fizz, fizz. Oh, what a relief it is.

___ 5. It keeps going and going . . .

___ 6. Can you hear me now?

___ 7. America's storyteller

___ 8. Away go troubles down the drain

___ 9. Nothin' says lovin' like somethin' from the oven.

___ 10. Sweet as the moment when the pod went "pop."

___ 11. Splash it all over.

___ 12. Where the rubber meets the road

___ 13. Not a cough in a carload

___ 14. The instrument of the immortals

___ 15. Put a tiger in your tank.

___ 16. Zoom, zoom, zoom

___ 17. Say it with flowers.

___ 18. Tastes so good, cats ask for it by name.

a. Brut after-shave

b. Meow Mix

c. Victor Talking Machine Co.

d. Kodak

e. Esso/Exxon

f. FTD (Interflora)

g. Steinway & Sons

h. Energizer

i. Firestone Tires

j. Timex

k. Alka-Seltzer

l. Verizon

m. Rice Krispies

n. Pillsbury

o. Old Gold Cigarettes

p. Birds Eye Peas

q. Mazda

r. Roto-Rooter

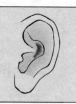

Slogans that Deal with Sound ANSWER SHEET

1.	His master's voice	c.	Victor Talking Machine Co.
2.	It takes a licking and keeps on ticking.	j.	Timex
3.	Snap, crackle, pop	m.	Rice Krispies
4.	Plop, plop, fizz, fizz. Oh, what a relief it is.	k.	Alka-Seltzer
5.	It keeps going and going . . .	h.	Energizer
6.	Can you hear me now?	l.	Verizon
7.	America's storyteller	d.	Kodak
8.	Away go troubles down the drain	r.	Roto-Rooter
9.	Nothin' says lovin' like somethin' from the oven.	n.	Pillsbury
10.	Sweet as the moment when the pod went "pop."	p.	Birds Eye Peas
11.	Splash it all over.	a.	Brut after-shave
12.	Where the rubber meets the road	i.	Firestone Tires
13.	Not a cough in a carload	o.	Old Gold Cigarettes
14.	The instrument of the immortals	g.	Steinway & Sons
15.	Put a tiger in your tank.	e.	Esso/Exxon
16.	Zoom, zoom, zoom	q.	Mazda
17.	Say it with flowers.	f.	FTD (Interflora)
18.	Tastes so good, cats ask for it by name.	b.	Meow Mix

FACILITATOR: *As you are reviewing the answers, have people imagine the sounds that the advertisers hope to elicit. What does ticking sound like? What would an instrument of an immortal sound like? What would rubber meeting the road sound like? Does thinking about the sounds increase one's desire to purchase the item?*

Things You Hear Outside

Oftentimes, we listen, but we don't really hear. We don't really pay attention to the sounds around us. Think about this fact as you complete the following activity. Sit quietly outside for 10–15 minutes, preferably with your eyes closed, paying very close attention to all of the sounds around you. Make a list of all of these sounds.

1.

2.

3.

4.

5.

6.

7.

8.

9.

10.

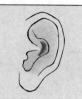

Airplanes flying overhead

Babies crying

Bags rustling

Bees buzzing

Bicycles riding by

Birds singing

Cars driving by

Cats meowing

Children playing

Church bells ringing

Clothes rustling

Dogs barking

Doors opening and closing

Flags flapping in the wind

Flies buzzing

Garbage trucks loading trash

Glasses clinking

Hammers pounding

Heart beating

Helicopters flying overhead

Horns honking

Ice cream trucks playing songs or ringing bells

Jackets zipping and unzipping

Leaves rustling

Pages of books, magazines, or papers turning

People eating and drinking

People shoveling

People skating

People speaking in foreign languages

People speaking with accents

People talking

Radios playing

Rain falling

Roosters crowing

Sirens blaring

Soft drink cans opening

Thunder roaring

Trains passing by

Water running

Whistles sounding

Wind blowing

FACILITATOR: *Ask participants to sit outside for 10–15 minutes, preferably in a park or other public place, and list all of the sounds they hear around them. Being present and paying close attention is one of the most important things we can teach people to enhance their memory. This exercise can teach participants to pay attention to what they hear, especially if they can block out visual and other distractions. Listed above are some sounds that you may use for discussion after participants have supplied as many answers as they can.*

Hearing and Emotions

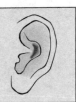

Your sense of hearing is powerfully related to your emotional memory. For example, what do you think of when you hear "The Star-Spangled Banner"? *Pride? Joy?* What about the sound of a train whistle? *Anticipation?* Listed below are common emotions. For this exercise, look at each emotion, and list sounds or things that you hear that make you feel that emotion. Be creative in thinking about sounds—use nature, music, people, animals, machines, and so forth. Share some of the memories that these sounds bring up.

1. Surprised *(example: balloon popping)*

2. Relaxed

3. Joyful

4. Amused

5. Awestruck

6. Fearful

7. Content

8. Gracious

9. In love

10. Proud

11. Cautious

12. Empowered

13. Peaceful

14. Inspired

15. Nervous

16. Excited

17. Hungry

Hearing and Emotions ANSWER SHEET

1. Surprised — **Balloon popping, car horn honking**

2. Relaxed — **Bubbling creek, harp**

3. Joyful — **Kids playing**

4. Amused — **Comedian telling a joke, people laughing**

5. Awestruck — **Waves crashing**

6. Fearful — **Gunshots**

7. Content — **Family discussion**

8. Gracious — **Gospel music**

9. In love — **Romantic songs, wedding march**

10. Proud — **National anthem**

11. Cautious — **Scary movie music, thunder**

12. Empowered — **Trumpets**

13. Peaceful — **Heartbeat, rain falling**

14. Inspired — **Cheering, clapping**

15. Nervous — **Airplane engines, wolves howling**

16. Excited — **Starting gun**

17. Hungry — **Food sizzling, popcorn popping**

FACILITATOR: *The sense of hearing is important in memory. Years after an experience, hearing a certain sound can immediately bring up memories of the event. For example, take the roar of a crowd at a ballgame or the sound of kids in the schoolyard. As people age, hearing is an especially important component of healthy memory. If a person is experiencing hearing loss, he or she may have difficulty remembering things that are important. Therefore, if someone is experiencing memory problems, his or her hearing should be checked and, if needed, the person should be fitted for a hearing aid to ensure that his or her change in memory is not due to an inability to hear well.*

In this exercise, participants recall a sound that reminds them of a certain emotion. Encourage participants to be creative with their responses, and remind them that there are no right or wrong answers. For additional discussion, ask participants to name their favorite sounds, funny sounds, sounds that are annoying, sounds according to the seasons, or sounds that animals make. Some sounds that you can use for discussion are listed above.

Things with a Strong Smell

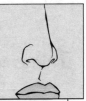

Using the letters of the alphabet, name as many items as you can that have a strong smell. In your mind, go through your kitchen, bathroom, garage, and other rooms, and then go outdoors to think of smells. A trip to the grocery store, whether imaginary or in person, may also help bring smells to mind.

A

B

C

D

E

F

G

H

I

J

K

L

M

N

O

P/Q

R

S

T

U/V

W

X/Y/Z

Things with a Strong Smell ANSWER SHEET

A	Acid, after-shave, alcohol, almond flavoring, ammonia, anise, aromatherapy
B	Bacon, bakeries, beer, bleach, broccoli, Brussels sprouts, burnt toast
C	Cabbage, catnip, cauliflower, cheese, chlorine, cigarettes, cigars, cinnamon, cloves, coffee
D	Deodorant, dill, dogs
E	Ether, eucalyptus, exhaust
F	Feet, fertilizer, fish, flowers
G	Garbage, garlic, gas, ginger
H	Hairspray, hay, honeysuckle, horseradish
I	Incense, insect spray, iodine
J	Jasmine, juices, junk food
K	Kelp, kerosene, ketchup
L	Lamb, lavender, lemon, licorice, Limburger cheese
M	Manure, marshland, mildew, mint, mold, mothballs
N	Nectarines, new cars, nutmeg
O	Olive oil, onions, oranges, ouzo
P/Q	Paint, paint thinner, pepper, peppermint, perfume, popcorn, potpourri, quince
R	Rosemary, roses, rotten eggs, rubber burning
S	Sage, skunk, smoke, soap
T	Tabasco, tar, thyme, tobacco, tuna, turpentine
U/V	Urine, vanilla, Vicks VapoRub, vinegar
W	Waste, wet wool, whiskey, wines, witch hazel
X/Y/Z	Yarrow, yeast, zoos

FACILITATOR: *After participants have listed as many items as possible, use clues regarding the above smells to jog their memories. Discuss whether or not the smells are good or bad, memorable or not, and so forth. Add other things to the list.*

Strengthen Your Mind by Einberger & Sellick. © 2007 by Health Professions Press, Inc.

Identification of Items by Smell

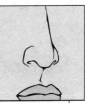

The sense of smell is very important in helping us to recall memories. Oftentimes, though, we don't really pay attention to the smells around us. Increase your sense of smell with the following exercise. Have a family member or facilitator of your group gather 10 distinct-smelling items and place them in separate bags. Without looking at the items, put your nose near each bag. Smell the item and identify it. Write your answers below.

1.

2.

3.

4.

5.

6.

7.

8.

9.

10.

Identification of Items by Smell ANSWER SHEET

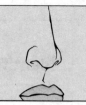

Almond flavoring	Jasmine
Bay leaves	Lavender
Blue cheese	Mint
Chocolate	Mothballs
Cinnamon	Mustard
Citrus fruit	Olive oil
Cloves	Popcorn
Coffee	Rose petals
Fish	Rosemary
Fragrant flowers	Tuna
Garlic	Vanilla
Horseradish	Vinegar

FACILITATOR: *Gather 10 of the above items and place them in separate bags. Make sure that the smells are very strong and, therefore, easy to identify. Ask participants to name each item as you pass the bags around. Ask the following questions: Which smell did you like the most? The least? Why are these smells memorable? Do you have suggestions for other items that would be identifiable by smell alone?*

Description of Smells

We encounter many smells in our everyday lives, from cookies baking to fresh fertilizer in the garden. Think of words (e.g., pungent) that you can use to describe the different smells you encounter every day. As you do this activity, visualize yourself going through a typical day. What's your favorite morning smell? Which words could you use to describe it?

1.

2.

3.

4.

5.

6.

7.

8.

9.

10.

11.

12.

Description of Smells ANSWER SHEET

Awful	Musty
Bitter	Nasty
Burnt	Off
Clean	Pleasant
Dirty	Pungent
Fishy	Putrid
Foul	Rancid
Fragrant	Rotten
Fresh	Sour
Gaseous	Stale
Grassy	Strong
Greasy	Sweet
Great	Unforgettable
Mildewy	Unmistakable
Moldy	Yeasty

FACILITATOR: *After participants have had the opportunity to list as many one-word descriptions as they can think of having to do with smell, suggest the words above or give clues in an attempt to encourage participants to guess each adjective. Ask for an example of an item whose smell may fit each description. As you complete this exercise with them, it may be helpful to "take a journey" through the day along with them.*

Strengthen Your Mind by Einberger & Sellick. © 2007 by Health Professions Press, Inc.

Slogans that Deal with Taste

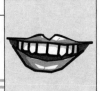

Slogans have been used for more than 100 years to increase familiarity with products and to lure customers to buy particular products. Some have been successful. Others have not. Each of the slogans below deals with the sense of taste. Can you match the slogan on the left with the product on the right?

___ 1. Tastes great. Less filling.

___ 2. Good to the last drop

___ 3. Betcha can't eat just one!

___ 4. The pause that refreshes

___ 5. Breakfast of champions

___ 6. Dangerously cheesy!

___ 7. Where's the beef?

___ 8. I can't believe I ate the whole thing.

___ 9. M'm M'm good

___ 10. They're grrreat!

___ 11. _____ tastes good, like a cigarette should.

___ 12. Everything's better with _____ on it.

___ 13. Brewed with pure Rocky Mountain spring water.

___ 14. The best part of waking up is _____ in your cup.

___ 15. America's most favorite dessert.

___ 16. The great American chocolate bar

___ 17. Come to where the flavor is.

___ 18. Double your pleasure, double your fun.

a. Doublemint

b. Marlboro

c. Wheaties

d. Folgers

e. Wendy's

f. Coca-Cola

g. Campbell's soup

h. Maxwell House

i. Miller Lite

j. Winston

k. Hershey's

l. Lay's potato chips

m. Kellogg's Frosted Flakes

n. Alka-Seltzer

o. Cheetos

p. Blue Bonnet

q. Jell-O

r. Coors

Slogans that Deal with Taste ANSWER SHEET

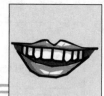

1. Tastes great. Less filling.

2. Good to the last drop

3. Betcha can't eat just one!

4. The pause that refreshes

5. Breakfast of champions

6. Dangerously cheesy!

7. Where's the beef?

8. I can't believe I ate the whole thing.

9. M'm M'm good

10. They're grrreat!

11. _____ tastes good, like a cigarette should.

12. Everything's better with _____ on it.

13. Brewed with pure Rocky Mountain spring water.

14. The best part of waking up is _____ in your cup.

15. America's most favorite dessert.

16. The great American chocolate bar

17. Come to where the flavor is.

18. Double your pleasure, double your fun.

i. **Miller Lite**

h. **Maxwell House**

l. **Lay's potato chips**

f. **Coca-Cola**

c. **Wheaties**

o. **Cheetos**

e. **Wendy's**

n. **Alka-Seltzer**

g. **Campbell's soup**

m. **Kellogg's Frosted Flakes**

j. **Winston**

p. **Blue Bonnet**

r. **Coors**

d. **Folgers**

q. **Jell-O**

k. **Hershey's**

b. **Marlboro**

a. **Doublemint**

FACILITATOR: *Once participants have finished, you may want to ask them if they have any other examples. Have they bought these products? Do they think advertising slogans such as these make a difference in whether or not people purchase these particular items? Have they tasted these products, and, if so, do they have any memories of the taste?*

Identification of Items by Taste

The sense of taste is the weakest of the five senses. As we get older, our taste buds become even less sensitive. This accounts for the fact that we often choose to eat foods that have a stronger taste or we add more seasonings to food in an attempt to make it "tastier" as we age. In the following exercise, pay special attention to how certain items taste, using only your sense of taste. Have a family member or the facilitator of your group place five distinct-tasting beverages (all without pulp) in small cups. Taste each one without looking at or smelling it. Write your answers below.

1.

2.

3.

4.

5.

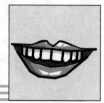

Chocolate milk (sweet)

Cranberry juice (sweet)

Grape juice (sweet)

Lemonade without pulp (sweet or sour depending on the sugar content)

Orange juice without pulp (sweet)

V-8 juice (salty)

Water with salt added (salty)

Grapefruit juice watered down (sour)

Water with lemon (sour)

Strong coffee (bitter)

Unsweetened iced tea (bitter)

FACILITATOR: *There are four basic tastes: sweet, salty, sour, and bitter. (Another one describing the meat taste is sometimes added.) Try the beverage taste test, using some of the above suggestions. Be sure to ask people not to look at or smell the drinks. Try to use at least one drink that provides each of the four different tastes.*

Once participants have completed the taste test, you might also want to try a couple more experiments. People are sure to enjoy an ice cream taste test, again without looking or smelling. Try to find ice cream that doesn't have chunks of fruit, nuts, and so forth in it. If you are unable to do so, you might want to explain that these items also allow us to use our sense of touch, giving us more clues.

Another taste test involves chunks of fruit (e.g., apples, pears, peaches, kiwi) on toothpicks. The textures will enable people to use the sense of touch, but taste is still the primary sense used. Although the ice cream and fruit taste tests don't take into account each of the four different tastes, they do allow participants to try to differentiate between the tastes of different items. And, of course, the taste tests are fun and provide for a great deal of conversation!

Taste Trivia

Taste is a fun sense to discuss! Below are questions and facts related to the sense of taste. Read the question and write the answer in the space provided.

1. You have about 10,000 of what item located on your tongue that helps you taste food?

2. Which taste is also known as the taste of acids and will make you pucker when you experience it?

3. What sticky, sweet addition to many foods is made by bees?

4. Too much of foods that have what taste can cause high blood pressure?

5. Many naturally occurring poisons have what taste?

6. Which sour fruit can be used to make pies and is also popular for flavoring beverages?

7. Which type of lettuce, often used in salads, is bitter and curly?

8. Which salty sauce is used for cooking in many Chinese dishes?

9. If you don't add cream and sugar to your morning coffee, many people would say that it has what taste?

10. Which taste is by far the most popular, especially among children?

11. What is the name of the recently determined fifth taste? (*Hint:* Although difficult to describe, it is commonly referred to as the taste associated with MSG.)

12. What sour cucumbers do many people like to put on hamburgers or eat straight out of the jar?

13. Which artificial sweetener was accidentally invented in 1878 and made public in 1900?

14. Which bitter fruit is the size of a softball and is most often grown in Florida?

15. Which sour vegetable is sometimes mistaken for a fruit and is most commonly used to make pies?

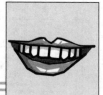

1. You have about 10,000 of what item on your tongue that helps you taste food?
   Taste buds

2. Which taste is also known as the taste of acid and will make you pucker when you experience it?
   Sour

3. What sticky, sweet addition to many foods is made by bees?
   Honey

4. Too much of foods that have what taste can cause high blood pressure?
   Salty

5. Many naturally occurring poisons have what taste?
   Bitter

6. Which sour fruit can be used to make pies and is also popular for flavoring beverages?
   Lemon

7. Which type of lettuce, often used in salads, is bitter and curly?
   Endive

8. Which salty sauce is used for cooking in many Chinese dishes?
   Soy sauce

9. If you don't add cream and sugar to your morning coffee, many people would say that it has what taste?
   Bitter

10. Which taste is by far the most popular, especially among children?
    Sweet

11. What is the name of the recently determined fifth taste? (*Hint:* Although difficult to describe, it is commonly referred to as the taste associated with MSG.)
    Umami

12. What sour cucumbers do many people like to put on hamburgers or eat straight out of the jar?
    Pickles

13. Which artificial sweetener was accidentally invented in 1878 and made public in 1900?
    Saccharin (or Sweet'N Low)

14. Which bitter fruit is the size of a softball and is most often grown in Florida?
    Grapefruit

15. Which sour vegetable is sometimes mistaken for a fruit and is most commonly used to make pies?
    Rhubarb

FACILITATOR: *For further activities related to taste, ask participants to make an A-to-Z list of all of the sweet foods they can think of. Then, do an A-to-Z list for each of the other tastes. Remind participants that they are challenging and strengthening their minds when they think creatively in this manner. Look up information on the fifth taste, umami, and ask participants if they agree that a fifth taste exists. Why or why not?*

Slogans that Deal with Touch

Each of the following slogans deals with the sense of touch, in one way or another. Imagine the feeling or touch described as you read each slogan. Match the slogan on the left with the name of the product that it advertises on the right.

___ 1. Reach out and touch someone.

___ 2. When it rains, it pours.

___ 3. A little dab'll do ya.

___ 4. Let your fingers do the walking.

___ 5. The milk chocolate melts in your mouth—not in your hand.

___ 6. Sometimes you feel like a nut.

___ 7. Look sharp, feel sharp, be sharp.

___ 8. Finger-lickin' good

___ 9. Please don't squeeze the _____.

___ 10. The quicker picker-upper

___ 11. You're in good hands with _____.

___ 12. That frosty mug sensation

___ 13. It's such a comfort to travel by bus—and leave the driving to us.

___ 14. When you need it the most

___ 15. No more tears

___ 16. Oh, what a feeling!

___ 17. If it feels good, then just do it.

___ 18. So creamy, it's almost fattening

a. Greyhound

b. Burma Shave

c. Gillette

d. AT&T

e. Jergens

f. Toyota

g. Nike

h. Morton Salt

i. Johnson's Baby Shampoo

j. A & W Root Beer

k. Brylcreem

l. Peter Paul Almond Joy

m. Allstate

n. Yellow Pages

o. M&M's

p. Bounty

q. Kentucky Fried Chicken

r. Charmin

Slogans that Deal with Touch ANSWER SHEET

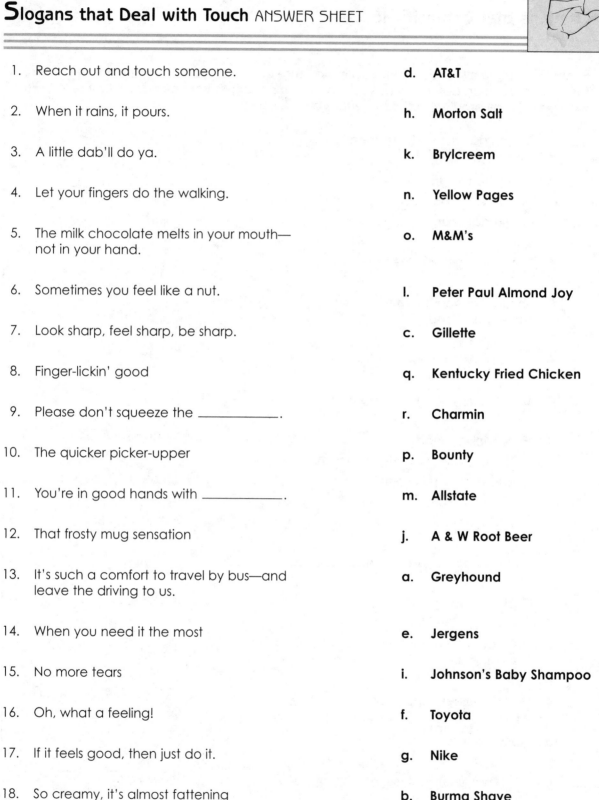

1. Reach out and touch someone.   d. **AT&T**

2. When it rains, it pours.   h. **Morton Salt**

3. A little dab'll do ya.   k. **Brylcreem**

4. Let your fingers do the walking.   n. **Yellow Pages**

5. The milk chocolate melts in your mouth—
    not in your hand.   o. **M&M's**

6. Sometimes you feel like a nut.   l. **Peter Paul Almond Joy**

7. Look sharp, feel sharp, be sharp.   c. **Gillette**

8. Finger-lickin' good   q. **Kentucky Fried Chicken**

9. Please don't squeeze the _____.   r. **Charmin**

10. The quicker picker-upper   p. **Bounty**

11. You're in good hands with _____.   m. **Allstate**

12. That frosty mug sensation   j. **A & W Root Beer**

13. It's such a comfort to travel by bus—and
    leave the driving to us.   a. **Greyhound**

14. When you need it the most   e. **Jergens**

15. No more tears   i. **Johnson's Baby Shampoo**

16. Oh, what a feeling!   f. **Toyota**

17. If it feels good, then just do it.   g. **Nike**

18. So creamy, it's almost fattening   b. **Burma Shave**

FACILITATOR: *After completing as much of this page as possible, ask participants to envision these phrases in their minds. Ask them the following questions: Do the visual images make sense? Do they make people want to buy or use the product? Are these slogans still used today, and, if not, would they still be effective if they were used now? Are there other companies that advertise using the sense of touch in their slogans?*

Identification of Items by Touch

Very often, we touch or hold things without really thinking about how they feel. Increase your sense of touch with the following exercise. Have a family member or the facilitator of your group gather 10 distinct-feeling items and place them in separate bags. Without looking at the items, reach in each bag. Touch and feel the item, and identify it. Write your answers below.

1.

2.

3.

4.

5.

6.

7.

8.

9.

10.

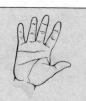

Bottle of glue	Nuts
Bows	Nuts and bolts
CD	Old-fashioned eraser
Cloves	Paper clips
Coins	Pine cone
Comb	Rice
Cotton balls	Rubber bands
Envelope	Sandpaper
Feathers	Shells
Glove	Sock
Key	Spools of thread
Leaf	Straw
Marshmallows	Sunflower seeds
Nail file	Toothbrush

FACILITATOR: *Even though our earliest memories are created through the sense of touch, we don't use this sense as much as we grow older. Therefore, it's especially important that we help those with early memory loss to strengthen their sense of touch so that they have one more tool to aid their memory. Gather multiple examples of 10 of the above items, and put each item in its own paper bag. Create a set of 10 bags for each participant. If you prefer, you can instead create one set of paper bags to pass around the group. Ask participants to identify the items simply by touching and feeling them. (No peeking!)*

Description of Items by Touch

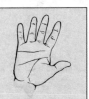

Imagine that you are touching different items and trying to describe how they feel. Mentally pick up some of these items and turn them over in your hands. Be aware of how they feel. List all of the words (e.g., rough) that you can think of that describe how items feel.

1.

2.

3.

4.

5.

6.

7.

8.

9.

10.

11.

12.

13.

14.

15.

Description of Items by Touch ANSWER SHEET

Abrasive	Light
Biting	Lumpy
Bumpy	Moist
Clammy	Oily
Coarse	Porous
Cold	Prickly
Crisp	Rigid
Dry	Rough
Dull	Rubbery
Fine	Sandy
Flaky	Scaly
Flexible	Scratchy
Fluffy	Sharp
Furry	Silky
Fuzzy	Slimy
Gooey	Slippery
Greasy	Smooth
Gritty	Soft
Hard	Sticky
Heavy	Velvety
Hot	Warm
Humid	Wet
Icy	

FACILITATOR: *After participants have listed all of the words that they can think of that describe how different items feel, give clues for the descriptions above that they haven't yet named. As an extension of this activity, ask them to name an item that would feel like this.*

Strengthen Your Mind by Einberger & Sellick. © 2007 by Health Professions Press, Inc.

Slogans that Deal with Vision

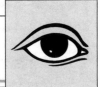

Each of the following slogans deals with the sense of vision. As you read the slogan, you may envision the product, especially if you have seen the advertisement on television or in a magazine. Match the slogans on the left with the products on the right.

___ 1. Ring around the collar

___ 2. You'll wonder where the yellow went.

___ 3. Fly the friendly skies.

___ 4. Does she or doesn't she?

___ 5. Look, Ma, no cavities!

___ 6. See America and see level.

___ 7. For virtually spotless dishes

___ 8. See the USA in your _____.

___ 9. Ask any mermaid you happen to see, "What's the best tuna?"

___ 10. We'll leave the light on for you.

___ 11. From the Land of Sky Blue Waters

___ 12. You've come a long way, Baby!

___ 13. Gets the red out

___ 14. You, too, can have a body like mine.

___ 15. It cleans your breath while it cleans your teeth.

___ 16. Look sharp, feel sharp, be sharp.

a. Charles Atlas

b. Chevrolet

c. Motel 6

d. Wisk

e. Gillette

f. Clairol

g. Visine

h. Pepsodent

i. Colgate

j. Cascade

k. United

l. Virginia Slims

m. Crest

n. Amtrak

o. Chicken of the Sea

p. Hamm's Beer

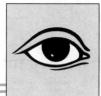

1. Ring around the collar   d. **Wisk**

2. You'll wonder where the yellow went.   h. **Pepsodent**

3. Fly the friendly skies.   k. **United**

4. Does she or doesn't she?   f. **Clairol**

5. Look, Ma, no cavities!   m. **Crest**

6. See America and see level.   n. **Amtrak**

7. For virtually spotless dishes   j. **Cascade**

8. See the USA in your _____.   b. **Chevrolet**

9. Ask any mermaid you happen to see, "What's the   o. **Chicken of the Sea**
    best tuna?"

10. We'll leave the light on for you.   c. **Motel 6**

11. From the Land of Sky Blue Waters   p. **Hamm's Beer**

12. You've come a long way, Baby!   l. **Virginia Slims**

13. Gets the red out   g. **Visine**

14. You, too, can have a body like mine.   a. **Charles Atlas**

15. It cleans your breath while it cleans your teeth.   i. **Colgate**

16. Look sharp, feel sharp, be sharp.   e. **Gillette**

FACILITATOR: *Once participants have completed this activity, ask for other examples and discuss the particular products. Do these slogans make a difference in whether or not participants would buy the products? Name a variety of other products and ask participants to think of slogans to advertise each item, using something to entice potential buyers visually.*

Strengthen Your Mind by Einberger & Sellick. © 2007 by Health Professions Press, Inc.

The Art of Observation

Oftentimes, we look at things, but we don't really see them. We don't really observe them in a conscious way. This activity will help you to better understand the art of observation. Imagine that you step out your front door and onto the edge of the street. Answer the following.

1. What color is the house or building across the street?

2. What color is the house or building next door?

3. How many houses or buildings are there on your block?

4. How many houses or buildings are there between your home and the corner?

5. Are telephone lines overhead or below ground?

6. Are there sidewalks on both sides of the street?

7. Are the sidewalks smooth or full of cracks?

8. Where is the closest streetlight?

9. What kinds of flowers do your next-door neighbors have in front of their home?

10. Do any of your neighbors have American flags hanging outside?

11. Have any of your neighbors decorated for the next holiday?

12. Do any of your neighbors have Christmas lights up?

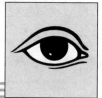

Answers to this worksheet will vary. For individuals who live in an assisted-living facility or who are unable to complete this exercise for some other reason, modify the activity as needed using an indoor area.

FACILITATOR: *This activity is great at pointing out the importance of observation in terms of memory. The more we concentrate on how things look, the more memorable these things become. Once participants have completed this worksheet, suggest that they take a walk down the street and pay close attention to everything they see. Then, ask them to return home and complete the activity again. Are they surprised at how much more they remember? Point out that the art of observation is always important and has great potential for enhancing our memory of things on our street, of people's names, of places we've been, of where our car is parked, and much more.*

A follow-up activity is to have participants close their eyes. Then, ask them to describe in as much detail as possible the room they are in and all of its details.

1. *What color(s) are the walls? The floors?*

2. *Are the walls smooth or textured?*

3. *Are there pictures on the wall?*

4. *Where are the light switches?*

5. *What color are the chairs?*

6. *What materials are they made from?*

7. *How many windows are there?*

Again, point out the art of observation and how important it is to help us remember things.

Another activity is for participants to go on a walk outside and, upon returning, list everything they have seen. This is great to do as a group as we all tend to notice different things.

Strengthen Your Mind by Einberger & Sellick. © 2007 by Health Professions Press, Inc.

Vision and Memory

Our sense of sight is one of the most important senses that we use in everyday life. It is also important in memory; things that we really focus on are easier to remember. For this exercise, think of a time when you have been in each of the following environments, and list answers to questions a through d below. If there are any settings listed that you have not experienced, use your imagination, and think of what you might see if you were there.

a.   Name something that is red.
b.   Name a person whom you would see.
c.   Name something that is on wheels.
d   Name something that is rectangular.

1.   At the Thanksgiving table:
     a.
     b.
     c.
     d.

2.   At a football game:
     a.
     b.
     c.
     d.

3.   In a classroom:
     a.
     b.
     c.
     d.

4.   In a vegetable garden:
     a.
     b.
     c.
     d.

5.   On a camping trip:
     a.
     b.
     c.
     d.

Vision and Memory ANSWER SHEET

a. Name something that is red.
b. Name a person whom you would see.
c. Name something that is on wheels.
d. Name something that is rectangular.

1. At the Thanksgiving table:
   a. **Cherry pie, cranberry sauce, red wine, tablecloth**
   b. **Pilgrims, relatives**
   c. **Food cart**
   d. **Candleholder, serving tray, stick of butter**

2. At a football game:
   a. **Flag, ketchup, seats, uniform**
   b. **Fans, the media, players, referee**
   c. **Cameras, cars in parking lot, vending machines**
   d. **Scoreboard, seat**

3. In a classroom:
   a. **Apple, color chart**
   b. **Room helper, students, teacher**
   c. **Overhead projector on cart, television on cart**
   d. **Book, chalkboard, desk**

4. In a vegetable garden:
   a. **Ladybugs, strawberries, tomatoes**
   b. **Chef, gardener, exterminator**
   c. **Hose reel, sprayer**
   d. **Garden box, hoe, trellis**

5. On a camping trip:
   a. **Blanket, bug bites, cooler, thermos**
   b. **Family, friends, park ranger**
   c. **Boat trailer, camper, car, cooler, grill, recreational vehicle (RV)**
   d. **Blanket, pillow, sleeping bag, tackle box, tent bottom**

FACILITATOR: *This is a great activity to encourage people to use their creativity. There are no right or wrong answers. Rather, the benefit for participants lies in challenging their brains to think abstractly. To elaborate on this activity, ask additional questions and add more scenarios. Or, ask each participant to contribute a scenario. Encourage participants to share their answers and the stories that they remember. After everyone has shared, use the above answers for further discussion.*

 Strengthen Your Mind by Einberger & Sellick. © 2007 by Health Professions Press, Inc.

Grocery Store Scavenger Hunt

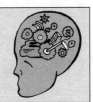

Grocery stores can be a great place to use all your senses. Take a trip to your local grocery store to identify the following items. If this is not possible, use magazines, newspapers, or simply your imagination to complete the exercise. Whichever way you do it, you're sure to bring up many memories associated with food!

1. Name two items (e.g., clove of garlic) that you could identify by feel alone.

2. Name two items that have a sour taste.

3. Name two items (e.g., lemon) that you could identify by smell without having to see them.

4. Name two items—not in the produce section—that are red.

5. Name two items that are soft.

6. Name two items that make a fairly loud noise when eaten.

7. Name two fruits that have a strong smell.

8. Name two vegetables that have a strong smell.

9. Name two items that are sticky (in or out of the package).

Grocery Store Scavenger Hunt ANSWER SHEET

1. Name two items (e.g., clove of garlic) that you could identify by feel alone.
   Bananas, eggs, hot dogs/sausage, spaghetti

2. Name two items that have a sour taste.
   Lemon, lime, sour cream, vinegar

3. Name two items (e.g., lemon) that you could identify by smell without having to see them.
   Bleach, chocolate, citrus fruits, coffee, fish, herbs and spices, Limburger cheese

4. Name two items—not in the produce section—that are red.
   Canned beets, ketchup, Red Hots candy, red licorice, sweet and sour sauce, tomato sauce

5. Name two items that are soft.
   Bread, cotton balls, baked goods, marshmallows, toilet paper, Twinkies

6. Name two items that make a fairly loud noise when eaten.
   Bubble gum, carrots, celery, crackers, croutons, hard candy, potato chips

7. Name two fruits that have a strong smell.
   Bananas, citrus fruits, strawberries

8. Name two vegetables that have a strong smell
   Cabbage, onions, peppers

9. Name two items that are sticky (in or out of the package).
   Cinnamon rolls, jams and jellies, molasses, sticky buns, syrup

FACILITATOR: *This scavenger hunt could be done individually, in small groups, or in one large group. It is a good activity to use after going through each of the senses individually in order to explain to participants how important it is that we use ALL of our senses to enhance our memory. Above are a few sample answers to get the conversation started.*

Strengthen Your Mind by Einberger & Sellick. © 2007 by Health Professions Press, Inc.

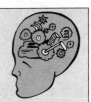

Tying It All Together

In this exercise, you will stimulate all of your senses by looking at pictures in magazines, newspapers, or other printed materials. You will pick five pictures and use your imagination to describe what you think your senses would detect if you were in the situations illustrated in the pictures. Be creative, and don't be afraid to close your eyes and imagine yourself in each picture. This will help to stimulate each of your senses so that you can describe what you perceive.

1. **Touch:** Find a picture in which you would feel cold or wet.

    Taste: What would you want to eat or drink in this situation?

    Smell: What would the air smell like?

    Hearing: What sounds would you hear?

    Vision: What or who might you see?

2. **Taste:** Find a picture that shows food that would taste sweet and sugary.

    Smell: What would the air smell like in this situation?

    Hearing: What sounds would you hear?

    Vision: What or who might you see?

    Touch: What would the food in the picture feel like?

3. **Smell:** Find a picture in which the air would smell clean and fresh.

    Hearing: What sounds would you hear in this situation?

    Vision: What or who might you see?

    Touch: Pick an item in the picture. What would it feel like?

    Taste: What would you want to eat or drink in this situation?

4. **Hearing:** Find a picture in which you would hear loud cheering.

    Vision: What or who might you see in this situation?

    Touch: Pick an item in the picture. What would it feel like?

    Taste: What would you want to eat or drink in this situation?

    Smell: What would the air smell like in the picture?

5. **Vision:** Find a picture of a place that you would like to visit on vacation.

    Touch: Pick an item in the picture. What would it feel like?

    Taste: What would you want to eat or drink in this situation?

    Smell: What would the air smell like in the picture?

    Hearing: What sounds would you hear in this situation?

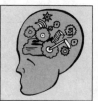

1. Touch: **Picture of a child playing in the rain**
    Taste: **Warm cup of hot chocolate or coffee**
    Smell: **Great smell of rain**
    Hearing: **Ping of the raindrops hitting the rooftop, the umbrella, and the ground**
    Vision: **Other people walking or running in the rain**

2. Taste: **Picture of a candy bar**
    Smell: **Wonderful, sweet smell of chocolate**
    Hearing: **Crinkle of the candy wrapper**
    Vision: **Colorful candy wrapper**
    Touch: **Smooth, sticky**

3. Smell: **Picture of laundry detergent**
    Hearing: **Woosh of the washing machine**
    Vision: **Basket full of clean clothes**
    Touch: **Fluffy, soft (towels)**
    Taste: **Salty junk food (eaten while waiting for washing machine to finish)**

4. Hearing: **Picture of a baseball game**
    Vision: **Child at his first little league game**
    Touch: **Hard bleacher seats**
    Taste: **Sugary cotton candy**
    Smell: **Popcorn and hot dogs**

5. Vision: **Picture of a couple in a gondola in Venice**
    Touch: **Cold chill of water**
    Taste: **Pasta**
    Smell: **Salty**
    Hearing: **Swoosh of paddle going through the water**

FACILITATOR: The five senses can be stimulated in a variety of ways. This activity is one suggestion. The above scenarios are just examples of what people may find in magazines. Ask participants to share their answers with one another. Invite them to offer ideas for other participants' pictures. Discuss how important it is to use all of our senses, not just seeing and hearing, to maximize our memory. Ask participants for suggestions of activities that involve all of the senses.

An Imaginary Journey of Your Senses

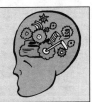

Take an imaginary journey to your favorite place. "Sit" for a while and discover your surroundings. *Look* at all that's around you. *Touch* those things most appealing to you. *Smell* items you believe may have a wonderful or memorable smell. *Listen* to all of the sounds. Imagine what things would *taste* like. Celebrate your senses! List two items you encountered on your journey in each of the following categories.

1. Listen
   a.
   b.

2. Look
   a.
   b.

3. Smell
   a.
   b.

4. Taste
   a.
   b.

5. Touch
   a.
   b.

An Imaginary Journey of Your Senses ANSWER SHEET

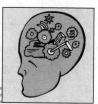

1. Listen
   a. **Water pouring over the rocks**
   b. **Birds chirping**

2. Look
   a. **Sticks floating down the stream**
   b. **Mountains in the distance**

3. Smell
   a. **Clean air**
   b. **Flowers in bloom**

4. Taste
   a. **The fish that you catch and fry on the grill**
   b. **The greens Native Americans may have eaten**

5. Touch
   a. **The feathery ferns surrounding the stream**
   b. **The slippery rocks underfoot as you cross the stream**

FACILITATOR: *Answers on this worksheet will vary as people take different journeys. As an example, one may take a journey to a nearby stream, in which case the above answers could be given as examples.*

After you've finished this activity and participants have had a chance to share their answers, discuss the importance of taking in all that's around us to "maximize" our memories. Point out that the more senses we use to remember something, the greater the likelihood that we will remember it.

A-to-Z Worksheets

Now that you have learned about, and stimulated, your senses, you will have the opportunity to complete more worksheets based on a variety of subjects. Each letter of the alphabet has two worksheets with a topic that begins with that letter. For example, under the letter *A*, you will find the worksheets *Addresses, Streets, Highways, and Bridges* and *All About Automobiles.* You can go through the worksheets in alphabetical order or you can pick and choose them in any order you would like.

Taking time to complete the worksheets in this manual is one of the most beneficial things you can do for your mind. Challenging your mind on a daily basis can help you to sharpen your mental capabilities and stimulate your memory. The subjects in the following pages span generations and cultures. Although some of the answers may come easily to you, some may be more difficult. It will be helpful to have some of the following resources available while working:

- Other people—friends, family, relatives, and neighbors

- Encyclopedia

- Dictionary

- Internet

- Maps

If you get stumped, pick up the telephone and call a friend or just leave the answer blank—you will be able to find the answers on the back of the page. In addition to the answers, the back of the page will also give you ideas and/or suggestions for expanding the topic. There will also be a paragraph at the bottom of the page to give you, a friend, a family member, or the facilitator of your group ideas on how to do more with each activity.

Exploring the subjects of these worksheets is just the beginning. Once you are finished, there are hundreds more topics that you can create on your own. Choose a new word from the dictionary each day or learn more about a hobby or pastime that is a favorite. Above all, enjoy the time that you spend on the worksheets, and enlist the help of others to make the process even more fun. You will be surprised at how easily the conversation flows and new subjects arise. Throughout the process of looking for the answers, you will stimulate your mind, gain knowledge, and take a trip down memory lane. Enjoy!

Addresses, Streets, Highways, and Bridges

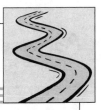

There are thousands of bridges and highways and innumerable streets and addresses throughout the world. Most are unknown except to the people who live nearby. The following places, though, are recognizable to many Americans and to some people in other parts of the world. Match the description on the left with the place on the right.

____ 1. The Prime Minister of England lives at this address.

____ 2. A "Christmas Miracle" took place on this street, according to a popular movie.

____ 3. This English bridge was moved from London to Arizona.

____ 4. Many people sit in cafes, shop at boutiques, or attend the cinema on this famous Parisian avenue.

____ 5. Big Bird, Oscar the Grouch, and Cookie Monster live on this street.

____ 6. The President of the United States lives at this address.

____ 7. This famous San Francisco bridge opened in 1937.

____ 8. This network of roads runs nearly the entire distance from Alaska to southern Chile, linking the Northern Hemisphere with the southern one.

____ 9. Sherlock Holmes lives at this address.

____ 10. This famous Chicago shopping district is on Michigan Avenue.

____ 11. This New York bridge was originally built for horse-drawn traffic and trolleys and was opened in 1883.

____ 12. This well-known street is located in the French Quarter in New Orleans.

____ 13. You can "get your kicks" on this historic highway that runs from Chicago to Los Angeles.

____ 14. This set of bridges in Thailand, popularized in a 1957 movie with William Holden, was assembled by prisoners.

____ 15. This television show debuted in 1958 and starred, among others, Kookie, who was always combing his hair.

a. *Bridge on the River Kwai*

b. Golden Gate Bridge

c. Brooklyn Bridge

d. 10 Downing Street

e. Champs-Élysées

f. Pan-American Highway

g. Route 66

h. Magnificent Mile

i. *77 Sunset Strip*

j. 34th Street

k. 1600 Pennsylvania Avenue

l. Bourbon Street

m. London Bridge

n. 221B Baker Street

o. Sesame Street

Addresses, Streets, Highways, and Bridges
ANSWER SHEET

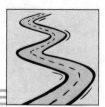

1. The Prime Minister of England lives at this address.

    d.   **10 Downing Street**

2. A "Christmas Miracle" took place on this street, according to a popular movie.

    j.   **34th Street**

3. This English bridge was moved from London to Arizona.

    m.   **London Bridge**

4. Many people sit in cafes, shop at boutiques, or attend the cinema on this famous Parisian avenue.

    e.   **Champs-Élysées**

5. Big Bird, Oscar the Grouch, and Cookie Monster live on this street.

    o.   **Sesame Street**

6. The President of the United States lives at this address.

    k.   **1600 Pennsylvania Avenue**

7. This famous San Francisco bridge opened in 1937.

    b.   **Golden Gate Bridge**

8. This network of roads runs nearly the entire distance from Alaska to southern Chile, linking the Northern Hemisphere with the southern one.

    f.   **Pan-American Highway**

9. Sherlock Holmes lives at this address.

    n.   **221B Baker Street**

10. This famous Chicago shopping district is on Michigan Avenue.

    h.   **Magnificent Mile**

11. This New York bridge was originally built for horse-drawn traffic and trolleys and was opened in 1883.

    c.   **Brooklyn Bridge**

12. This well-known street is located in the French Quarter in New Orleans.

    l.   **Bourbon Street**

13. You can "get your kicks" on this historic highway that runs from Chicago to Los Angeles.

    g.   **Route 66**

14. This set of bridges in Thailand, popularized in a 1957 movie with William Holden, was assembled by prisoners.

    a.   *Bridge on the River Kwai*

15. This television show debuted in 1958 and starred, among others, Kookie, who was always combing his hair.

    i.   *77 Sunset Strip*

FACILITATOR: *Some factual, some fictional, many of these famous bridges, addresses, streets, and highways are sure to be recognizable. For each place, ask participants who has been there, who would like to visit, and what they think made the place so famous. Ask for other suggestions of famous addresses and so forth. Would places like Haight-Ashbury in San Francisco or the Tower Bridge in London have been recognizable? Why or why not? Use a map.*

Strengthen Your Mind by Einberger & Sellick. © 2007 by Health Professions Press, Inc.

All About Automobiles

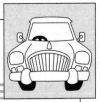

No single invention has changed American society as much as the automobile. Cars have become more and more efficient and safe, yet the early cars of the 1900s hold nostalgic memories for many. Answer the questions below to reminisce about older cars and learn about some of the newer ones.

1. Which two countries produce the most cars?

2. In 1876, who invented the first gas motor engine?

3. Which country is famous for its superhighways on which speeds often exceed 100 mph?

4. Name five American automakers.

5. Name five foreign automakers.

6. What does the phrase *pedal to the metal* mean?

7. What open addition to the back of many cars was also known as the "mother-in-law" seat?

8. What is the minimum age to earn a driver's license in most states?

9. What man popularized the gas-powered automobile and created an American automobile dynasty?

10. What famous Ford car was named after Henry Ford's only son and was originally known as the "E" car?

11. When first invented, automobiles were nicknamed what?

12. What type of open-air theater reached the height of popularity in the 1950s and was a popular destination for both families and teenagers?

13. Which automobile is known for its distinctive round shape? (*Hint*: Since its creation in the 1930s, more than 21 million have been produced.)

14. What famous automobile race, known as the "Superbowl of NASCAR," is 500 miles long and held each year in Florida?

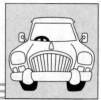

All About Automobiles ANSWER SHEET

1. Which two countries produce the most cars?
   Japan and United States

2. In 1876, who invented the first gas motor engine?
   Nicolaus August Otto

3. Which country is famous for its superhighways on which speeds often exceed 100 mph?
   Germany, the Autobahn

4. Name five American automakers.
   Buick, Cadillac, Chevrolet, Chrysler, Dodge, Ford, General Motors, Lincoln, Mercury, Oldsmobile, Saturn

5. Name five foreign automakers.
   BMW, Honda, Hyundai, Isuzu, Mazda, Mitsubishi, Nissan, Porsche, Toyota, Volkswagen

6. What does the phrase *pedal to the metal* mean?
   Go as fast as you can

7. What open addition to the back of many cars was also known as the "mother-in-law" seat?
   Rumble seat

8. What is the minimum age to earn a driver's license in most states?
   Sixteen

9. What man popularized the gas-powered automobile and created an American automobile dynasty?
   Henry Ford

10. What famous Ford car was named after Henry Ford's only son and was originally known as the "E" car?
    Edsel

11. When first invented, automobiles were nicknamed what?
    Horseless carriage

12. What type of open-air theater reached the height of popularity in the 1950s and was a popular destination for both families and teenagers?
    Drive-in theater

13. Which automobile is known for its distinctive round shape? (*Hint:* Since its creation in the 1930s, more than 21 million have been produced.)
    Volkswagen (VW) Beetle, or Bug

14. What famous automobile race, known as the "Superbowl of NASCAR," is 500 miles long and held each year in Florida?
    Daytona 500

FACILITATOR: *Cars bring up a variety of discussion topics. After participants complete the worksheet, encourage them to share using the following questions: What was your first car like? How old were you when you first learned to drive? What do you think about the way cars are made today versus the way they were made in the early- to mid-1900s? Can you name some of the most famous makes and models over the past 100 years? Do Americans have a love affair with the automobile? Why or why not?*

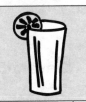

Beverages Throughout History

Americans drink a large variety of beverages. According to most reports, we drink more carbonated soft drinks than any other drink! Using the clues, name the beverage or thing associated with a beverage.

1. Napa Valley is most famous for what type of drink?

2. Name two sources, other than cows, from which milk can come.

3. Someone who drinks too much beer can be said to have what type of stomach?

4. Seattle is most famous for what type of drink?

5. Children all over the United States sell what drink at stands?

6. Name five brands of soft drinks.

7. Milwaukee is famous for what type of beverage?

8. Young men who served drinks and ice cream in a drugstore were often called what?

9. What wine made from rice is popular in Japan?

10. What dairy-based drink is popular at Christmas?

11. What was the name of the period during which the 18th Amendment forbid the sale of alcoholic beverages?

12. An undiluted fruit juice or a sweet liquid that attracts bees is called what?

13. What hot beverage is especially popular in England and China?

14. What is the best-selling beer in the world?

15. A soft drink, such as root beer, with ice cream added is called what?

16. According to many health experts, how much water should we drink each day?

17. A big marketing battle has existed for many years between which two cola products? (Which one do you like best?)

18. Puerto Rico is famous for producing what liquor?

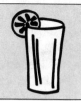

1. Napa Valley is most famous for what type of drink?
   Wine

2. Name two sources, other than cows, from which milk can come.
   Buffalo, camel, coconut, goat, sheep, soy

3. Someone who drinks too much beer can be said to have what type of stomach?
   Beer belly

4. Seattle is most famous for what type of drink?
   Coffee

5. Children all over the United States sell what drink at stands?
   Kool-Aid or lemonade

6. Name five brands of soft drinks.
   Barq's, Canada Dry, Coca-Cola, Dr Pepper, Fanta, Hires, Mountain Dew, Orangina, Pepsi, RC Cola, Seven-Up, Sprite

7. Milwaukee is famous for what type of beverage?
   Beer

8. Young men who served drinks and ice cream in a drugstore were often called what?
   Soda jerk

9. What wine made from rice is popular in Japan?
   Sake

10. What dairy-based drink is popular at Christmas?
    Eggnog

11. What was the name of the period during which the 18th Amendment forbid the sale of alcoholic beverages?
    Prohibition

12. An undiluted fruit juice or a sweet liquid that attracts bees is called what?
    Nectar

13. What hot beverage is especially popular in England and China?
    Tea

14. What is the best-selling beer in the world?
    Budweiser

15. A soft drink, such as root beer, with ice cream added is called what?
    Ice cream float

16. According to many health experts, how much water should we drink each day?
    8 glasses

17. A big marketing battle has existed for many years between which two cola products? (Which one do you like best?)
    Coca-Cola and Pepsi

18. Puerto Rico is famous for producing what liquor?
    Rum

FACILITATOR: *When reviewing the answers, try to have bottles, cans, or cartons of some of these beverages out on the table to increase visual awareness. Good discussion topics would include: What is everyone's favorite drink? Does anyone drink 8 glasses of water per day? Why is soda so popular? Did anyone ever have a Kool-Aid or lemonade stand when they were younger? Are certain drinks associated with particular occasions? Have participants try to name as many brand names as possible for certain beverages like beer.*

Books, Magazines, and Authors

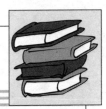

Whether you like to read classic novels or skim through popular magazines, reading is one of our favorite pastimes. Use this worksheet to learn more about the many authors and publications that are enjoyed around the world. Match the description of the book or author on the left with the answer on the right.

____ 1. With this weekly magazine that debuted in 1953 you can find your favorite television shows.

____ 2. This book by Mark Twain takes place on the Mississippi River.

____ 3. This magazine featured weekly illustrations by Norman Rockwell.

____ 4. This famous television talk show hostess is a great promoter of books and reading and has her own magazine.

____ 5. This book, divided into two sections, sold the most copies of any other book in history.

____ 6. These reference books are the largest selling of all print encyclopedias in the world.

____ 7. "Primers" featuring this boy and girl and their dog, Spot, were standard school texts from the 1930s to the 1960s.

____ 8. This Margaret Mitchell book was made into one of the most beloved films of all time.

____ 9. This children's book has made the phrase "I think I can" synonymous with optimism and the "can-do spirit."

____ 10. This red-and-white plaid cookbook is #1 in America today and has sold more than 32 million copies.

____ 11. This children's author is famous for his colorful works, including two of his most popular, *The Cat in the Hat* and *Green Eggs and Ham*.

____ 12. In 1930, this series of mystery books, popular with young women, debuted. The books starred a young woman as a detective who solved mysteries.

____ 13. A new edition of this book is published each year, featuring extreme record-breaking achievements.

____ 14. The home to most of this character's detective stories is 221B Baker Street.

____ 15. This book, featuring the ghosts of Christmas past, present, and future, is a favorite at the holidays.

a. *Better Homes and Gardens New Cook Book*

b. Sherlock Holmes

c. *The Bible*

d. *TV Guide*

e. Dr. Seuss

f. *A Christmas Carol*

g. *Gone with the Wind*

h. *The Little Engine That Could*

i. *Guinness World Records*

j. Nancy Drew

k. Oprah Winfrey

l. Dick and Jane

m. *The Adventures of Tom Sawyer*

n. *The Saturday Evening Post*

o. *World Book Encyclopedias*

Books, Magazines, and Authors ANSWER SHEET

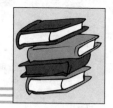

1. With this weekly magazine that debuted in 1953 you can find your favorite television shows.

   d. TV Guide

2. This book by Mark Twain takes place on the Mississippi River.

   m. The Adventures of Tom Sawyer

3. This magazine featured weekly illustrations by Norman Rockwell.

   n. The Saturday Evening Post

4. This famous television talk show hostess is a great promoter of books and reading and has her own magazine.

   k. Oprah Winfrey

5. This book, divided into two sections, sold the most copies of any other book in history.

   c. The Bible

6. These reference books are the largest selling of all print encyclopedias in the world.

   o. World Book Encyclopedias

7. "Primers" featuring this boy and girl and their dog, Spot, were standard school texts from the 1930s to the 1960s.

   l. Dick and Jane

8. This Margaret Mitchell book was made into one of the most beloved films of all time.

   g. Gone with the Wind

9. This children's book has made the phrase "I think I can" synonymous with optimism and the "can-do spirit."

   h. The Little Engine That Could

10. This red-and-white plaid cookbook is #1 in America today and has sold more than 32 million copies.

    a. Better Homes and Gardens New Cook Book

11. This children's author is famous for his colorful works, including two of his most popular, *The Cat in the Hat* and *Green Eggs and Ham.*

    e. Dr. Seuss

12. In 1930, this series of mystery books, popular with young women, debuted. The books starred a young woman as a detective who solved mysteries.

    j. Nancy Drew

13. A new edition of this book is published each year, featuring extreme record-breaking achievements.

    i. Guinness World Records

14. The home to most of this character's detective stories is 221B Baker Street.

    b. Sherlock Holmes

15. This book, featuring the ghosts of Christmas past, present, and future, is a favorite at the holidays.

    f. A Christmas Carol

FACILITATOR: *For further discussion, have the group brainstorm classic novels and writers. How do they compare to the popular books of today? Ask each person in the group to name his or her favorite book and why he or she likes it. Try to create an A-to-Z list of authors or classic novels. Has anyone in the group ever written a book or had an article published?*

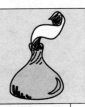

Chocolate, Chocolate, Chocolate

Chocolate is at the top of the list of favorite foods for millions of people. Recent research has shown that dark chocolate can have a positive effect on memory. Answer the following questions using your chocolate savvy!

1. What is chocolate made from?

2. In Hershey, Pennsylvania, what are the streetlights shaped like?

3. Which country consumes the most chocolate per person according to the Chocolate Manufacturers Association?

4. According to the slogan, who "makes the very best" chocolate?

5. Name five candy bars that contain chocolate.

6. In 1940, the Mars Company first sold what candy to soldiers going to World War II because it wouldn't melt in their hands?

7. Name three chocolate producers.

8. What is the most popular candy bar in the United States today, according to AskMen.com?

9. Name five items that are made from chocolate.

10. How much did a Hershey Bar cost in
    a. 1920?
    b. 1955?
    c. 1980?
    d. 2005?

11. Do more Americans prefer milk chocolate or dark? (How about you?)

12. What popular chocolate Easter egg comes from England?

13. Name two types of chocolate besides milk chocolate.

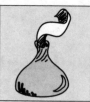

1. What is chocolate made from?
   Cocoa beans, seeds of the cacao tree

2. In Hershey, Pennsylvania, what are the streetlights shaped like?
   Hershey's Kisses

3. Which country consumes the most chocolate per person according to the Chocolate Manufacturers Association?
   Switzerland

4. According to the slogan, who "makes the very best" chocolate?
   Nestlé

5. Name five candy bars that contain chocolate.
   3Musketeers, Almond Joy, Butterfinger, Heath Toffee Bar, Hershey's Bar, Kit Kat, Mars, Milky Way, Mounds, Mr. Goodbar, Nestlé Crunch, Snickers, Twix, York Peppermint Pattie

6. In 1940, the Mars Company first sold what candy to soldiers going to World War II because it wouldn't melt in their hands?
   M&M'S

7. Name three chocolate producers.
   Baci, Baker's, Cadbury, Ghirardelli, Godiva, Guittard, Hershey's, Nestlé, Russell Stover, See's, Suchard, Toblerone, Whitman's

8. What is the most popular candy bar in the United States today, according to AskMen.com?
   Snickers

9. Name five items that are made from chocolate.
   Brownies, cake, candy, cookies, fudge, hot chocolate, pie, pudding, shakes, splits, sundaes, syrup

10. How much did a Hershey Bar cost in
    a. **3 cents in 1920**
    b. **5 cents in 1955**
    c. **25 cents in 1980**
    d. **approximately 75 cents in 2005**

11. Do more Americans prefer milk chocolate or dark? (How about you?)
    Milk chocolate—approximately 65% like milk chocolate best!

12. What popular chocolate Easter egg comes from England?
    Cadbury Creme Egg

13. Name two types of chocolate besides milk chocolate.
    Couverture, dark or bittersweet, semi-sweet, unsweetened or cocoa powder, white

FACILITATOR: *Chocolate is sure to be a lively topic for discussion. Ask each person for his or her favorite chocolate bar, favorite type of chocolate, favorite dessert with chocolate, and so forth. Ask for special memories associated with chocolate—a special Valentine's Day gift, an Easter egg, Halloween treats, and so forth. A fun and interesting activity to go along with this worksheet would be to have a taste test with different kinds of candy bars. Assemble a few different types of candy bars, cut them into small pieces, and have everyone guess the type. This could be done in a big group, small groups, or individually. Be sure to number each bar and pass out paper to each person, with numbered blanks to be filled in.*

Currencies from Around the World

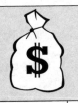

Whether you travel the world or explore your local hometown, exchanging money can be a mental workout. Use this worksheet to expand your knowledge of different currencies by writing the type of currency next to the country listed. (*Note:* Although most European countries now use the euro, list the type of currency each country used before being standardized.)

1. Switzerland

2. South Africa

3. Japan

4. China

5. Europe

6. United Kingdom

7. India

8. Germany

9. France

10. Italy

11. Mexico

12. Netherlands

13. Russia

14. Spain

15. Thailand

16. Vietnam

17. Canada

18. Argentina

19. Brazil

20. Croatia

Currencies from Around the World ANSWER SHEET

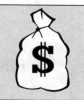

1. Switzerland   **Franc**

2. South Africa   **Rand**

3. Japan   **Yen**

4. China   **Yuan**

5. Europe   **Euro**

6. United Kingdom   **Pound**

7. India   **Rupee**

8. Germany   **Deutsche mark**

9. France   **Franc**

10. Italy   **Lira**

11. Mexico   **Peso**

12. Netherlands   **Guilder**

13. Russia   **Ruble**

14. Spain   **Pesetas**

15. Thailand   **Baht**

16. Vietnam   **Dong**

17. Canada   **Dollar**

18. Argentina   **Peso**

19. Brazil   **Real**

20. Croatia   **Kuna**

FACILITATOR: Use this exercise to encourage conversation about travel. Ask participants to name all of the countries that they have traveled to or lived in. What is it like to purchase goods with foreign money? For extra fun, look up exchange rates and compare the value of the dollar. Using a map would be helpful during this activity.

Desserts of Different Cultures

What a sweet way to exercise your mind! Many of these desserts from around the world can be found in our own supermarkets. Read the description on the left, and match it with the name of the treat on the right.

___ 1. This traditional Greek pastry is made with phyllo dough.

a. Gelato

___ 2. This Italian dessert is made with espresso coffee and ladyfingers.

b. Lebkuchen

___ 3. This dessert, often served in Spain or Mexico, is made of custard filling inside a baked pastry.

c. Biscotti

___ 4. This German Christmas cookie is usually honey flavored.

d. Anzac biscuits

___ 5. This holiday cookie is eaten by many Jewish families during Passover.

e. Baklava

___ 6. This versatile baked pudding is made in the French countryside.

f. Biscochitos

___ 7. This rich dessert was originally eaten by the poor in England to make use of stale bread.

g. Tiramisu

___ 8. This rich Italian ice cream is typically made with fresh fruit.

h. Apple pie

___ 9. This American dessert is made with apples, sugar, and cinnamon in a pastry crust.

i. Flan

___ 10. This traditional Australian cookie is named for the Australia-New Zealand Army Corps.

j. Rugelach

___ 11. These Mexican sugar cookies are usually enjoyed on Christmas Eve.

k. Clafouti

___ 12. This German sweet coffee cake is made with fruit and nuts.

l. Bread pudding

___ 13. This Jewish cookie is shaped like a crescent moon.

m. Pavlova

___ 14. These dense Italian cookies are used for dipping in coffee.

n. Macaroon

___ 15. This meringue-style dessert is named after a ballet dancer.

o. Kuchen

Desserts of Different Cultures ANSWER SHEET

1. This traditional Greek pastry is made with phyllo dough.

    e. Baklava

2. This Italian dessert is made with espresso coffee and ladyfingers.

    g. Tiramisu

3. This dessert, often served in Spain or Mexico, is made of custard filling inside a baked pastry.

    i. Flan

4. This German Christmas cookie is usually honey flavored.

    b. Lebkuchen

5. This holiday cookie is eaten by many Jewish families during Passover.

    n. Macaroon

6. This versatile baked pudding is made in the French countryside.

    k. Clafouti

7. This rich dessert was originally eaten by the poor in England to make use of stale bread.

    l. Bread pudding

8. This rich Italian ice cream is typically made with fresh fruit.

    a. Gelato

9. This American dessert is made with apples, sugar, and cinnamon in a pastry crust.

    h. Apple pie

10. This traditional Australian cookie is named for the Australia-New Zealand Army Corps.

    d. Anzac biscuits

11. These Mexican sugar cookies are usually enjoyed on Christmas Eve.

    f. Biscochitos

12. This German sweet coffee cake is made with fruit and nuts.

    o. Kuchen

13. This Jewish cookie is shaped like a crescent moon.

    j. Rugelach

14. These dense Italian cookies are used for dipping in coffee.

    c. Biscotti

15. This meringue-style dessert is named after a ballet dancer.

    m. Pavlova

FACILITATOR: *Encourage participants to share their favorite desserts and special times that the desserts were shared. Of the variety of desserts listed, how many have participants tried? As a bonus question, ask which of these sweets is the official state dessert of South Dakota. (Answer: Kuchen)*

    Strengthen Your Mind by Einberger & Sellick. © 2007 by Health Professions Press, Inc.

Dressings and Condiments

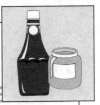

Sauces can make a bland dish wonderful! How could you use the following sauces in cooking? What types of foods would you put them on? For extra fun, name a specific brand that goes with each type of sauce.

Sauce	How it is used	Brand
1. Mayonnaise		
2. Mustard		
3. Ketchup		
4. Relish		
5. Teriyaki sauce		
6. Barbecue sauce		
7. Soy sauce		
8. Steak sauce		
9. Worcestershire sauce		
10. Pepper sauce		
11. Curry		
12. Hard sauce		
13. Salsa		
14. Fudge sauce		
15. Tomato sauce		
16. Pesto sauce		
17. Alfredo sauce		
18. Syrup		
19. Horseradish		

Dressings and Condiments ANSWER SHEET

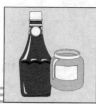

Sauce	How it is used	Brand
1. Mayonnaise	Egg salad, dips, potato salad, sandwiches, tuna fish	Best Foods, Hellmann's, Kraft, Miracle Whip
2. Mustard	Hamburgers, hot dogs, pretzels	Best Foods, Colman's, French's, Grey Poupon, Gulden's, Heinz
3. Ketchup	Eggs, French fries, hamburgers, hash browns	Del Monte, Heinz
4. Relish	Dressing, hot dogs, tartar sauce, Thousand Island	Del Monte, Heinz, Mezzetta, Mt. Olive, Vlasic
5. Teriyaki sauce	Chicken stir-fry, marinades, meats, rice, seafood	JES, Kikkoman, Soy Vay
6. Barbecue sauce	Chicken, dipping sauce for chicken nuggets, steak	Bullseye, Jack Daniel's, KC Masterpiece, Kraft, Sweet Baby Ray's, Tony Roma's
7. Soy sauce	Chow mein, rice, sauces, soups, stews, vegetables	Dynasty, Kikkoman, La Choy, Lee Kum Kee
8. Steak sauce	Meatloaf, meats	A1, Heinz 57, Lawry's, Lea and Perrins, Smith & Wollensky
9. Worcestershire sauce	Burgers, gravy, marinades, meatloaf	Lea and Perrins
10. Pepper sauce	Burritos, eggs, hash browns, pizza, salad	Crystal, Frank's, Tabasco
11. Curry	Chicken, potatoes, tofu, vegetables	S&B, Thai Kitchen
12. Hard sauce	Bread pudding, mincemeat pie, plum pudding	Crosse & Blackwell, Wilkin & Sons Ltd.
13. Salsa	Chips, fish, potatoes, salads	Arriba!, Herdez, La Victoria, Ortega, Pace
14. Fudge sauce	Cake, fondue, fruit, ice cream, milk	Hershey's, Mrs. Richardson's, Nestlé, Smucker's
15. Tomato sauce	Pasta, pizza, spaghetti	Bertolli, Classico, Contadina, Del Monte, Newman's Own, Prego, Ragú, S&W
16. Pesto sauce	Garlic bread, gnocchi, pasta	Buitoni, Monterey Pasta Company
17. Alfredo sauce	Fettuccine, lasagna	Bertolli, Buitoni, Classico, Ragú
18. Syrup	Crepes, pancakes, waffles	Aunt Jemima, Eggo, Hungry Jack, Log Cabin, Mrs. Butterworth's
19. Horseradish	Cocktail sauce, prime rib, sandwiches	Beaver, Mezzetta, Morehouse

FACILITATOR: *Most individuals have memories of cooking, whether in the kitchen or on the grill. This exercise will encourage participants to use their creative thinking skills to list all of the ways to use these types of sauces. Encourage participants to share their memories and ideas for how they used the different sauces they have listed.*

Strengthen Your Mind by Einberger & Sellick. © 2007 by Health Professions Press, Inc.

E.T. Phone Home—Famous Movie Lines

Talking motion pictures have been around more than 75 years. Thousands of movies have been made, featuring thousands of actors and actresses. Millions of lines have been said—some have made movie history. "E.T. phone home" is one of the most famous lines in recent years. It's from the movie *E.T.* The following lines were also said by a famous movie star in a famous movie. Name the star, character, and/or the movie.

1. "Elementary, my dear Watson."

2. "Frankly, my dear, I don't give a damn."

3. "When I'm good, I'm very good, but when I'm bad, I'm better."

4. "Here's looking at you, kid."

5. "Toto, I've a feeling we're not in Kansas anymore."

6. "I'll make him an offer he can't refuse."

7. "I'll be back."

8. "I don't know nothin 'bout birthin' babies."

9. "Of all the gin joints in all the towns in all the world, she walks into mine."

10. "Hey, STELLAAAAA!"

11. "What is it you want, Mary? What do you want? You want the moon? Just say the word, and I'll throw a lasso around it and pull it down."

12. "Gimme a whiskey, ginger ale on the side. And don't be stingy, baby."

13. "They call me *Mister* Tibbs."

14. "I coulda had class. I coulda been a contender."

15. "Well, here's another nice mess you've gotten me into."

E.T. Phone Home—Famous Movie Lines ANSWER SHEET

1. "Elementary, my dear Watson."
   Basil Rathbone as Sherlock Holmes, *The Adventures of Sherlock Holmes*

2. "Frankly, my dear, I don't give a damn."
   Clark Gable as Rhett Butler, *Gone with the Wind*

3. "When I'm good, I'm very good, but when I'm bad, I'm better."
   Mae West as Tira, *I'm No Angel*

4. "Here's looking at you, kid."
   Humphrey Bogart as Rick Blaine, *Casablanca*

5. "Toto, I've a feeling we're not in Kansas anymore."
   Judy Garland as Dorothy, *The Wizard of Oz*

6. "I'll make him an offer he can't refuse."
   Marlon Brando as Don Corleone or Al Pacino as Michael Corleone, *The Godfather*

7. "I'll be back."
   Arnold Schwarzenegger as The Terminator, *The Terminator*

8. "I don't know nothin 'bout birthin' babies."
   Butterfly McQueen as Prissy, *Gone with the Wind*

9. "Of all the gin joints in all the towns in all the world, she walks into mine."
   Humphrey Bogart as Rick Blaine, *Casablanca*

10. "Hey, STELLAAAAA!"
    Marlon Brando as Stanley Kowalski, *A Streetcar Named Desire*

11. "What is it you want, Mary? What do you want? You want the moon? Just say the word, and I'll throw a lasso around it and pull it down."
    Jimmy Stewart as George Bailey, *It's a Wonderful Life*

12. "Gimme a whiskey, ginger ale on the side. And don't be stingy, baby."
    Greta Garbo as Anna Christie, *Anna Christie*

13. "They call me *Mister* Tibbs."
    Sidney Poitier as Detective Virgil Tibbs, *In the Heat of the Night*

14. "I coulda had class. I coulda been a contender."
    Marlon Brando as Terry Malloy, *On the Waterfront*

15. "Well, here's another nice mess you've gotten me into."
    Oliver Hardy as himself, *Another Fine Mess* or *Sons of the Desert*

FACILITATOR: *As you review the answers, discuss each movie and its stars. Why are these lines memorable? Who has seen the movie? Did he or she like it? Were the stars famous for other movies? When did everyone first go to the movies? How much did it cost? What is each person's favorite movie ever? His or her favorite stars? How have movies changed through the years? Oftentimes, quotes are remembered differently by different people. Ask participants if there are any quotes that they remember as having other wordings (e.g., "Somehow, Toto, I don't think we're in Kansas anymore." "I'm gonna make him an offer he can't refuse." "When I'm good, I'm very, very good . . .").*

The *E*yes Have It

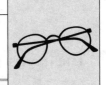

Our eyes are one of the most important parts of our bodies, and, as a result, a variety of expressions have popped up over the years that have the word eye in them. In addition, we use many objects in everyday life that are related to our sight. Read the questions below. Each answer has the word eye in it.

1. Something that is unpleasant to look at is called what?

2. Many women use what type of product to add color to their eyes?

3. What is a small hole in fabric for passing a needle called?

4. When two people agree or have the same opinion, it is said that they do what?

5. One of the two large pointed teeth in the upper jaw is called what?

6. Someone who sees something firsthand is called what?

7. When a person sees something that is a welcome sight, he or she might say that it is what?

8. What row of hairs grows above the eyes?

9. Name a traditional form of repayment or revenge.

10. What piece of material used to cover the eye is often worn by pirates?

11. To look directly at the eyes of someone is to make what?

12. What small device is used for administering medications?

13. What fringe of hairs grows along the edge of the eyes?

14. What portable lens is used to make objects appear larger?

15. To make efforts to get someone's attention is to try to do what?

16. To watch something very closely is to do what?

17. What is something that is striking, interesting, or attractive called?

18. Name an informal exclamation of disagreement.

The *E*yes Have It ANSWER SHEET

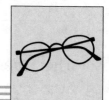

1. Something that is unpleasant to look at is called what?
    An eyesore

2. Many women use what type of product to add color to their eyes?
    Eye shadow or eyeliner

3. What is a small hole in fabric for passing a needle called?
    An eyelet

4. When two people agree or have the same opinion, it is said that they do what?
    See eye to eye

5. One of the two large pointed teeth in the upper jaw is called what?
    An eyetooth

6. Someone who sees something firsthand is called what?
    An eyewitness

7. When a person sees something that is a welcome sight, he or she might say that it is what?
    A sight for sore eyes

8. What row of hairs grows above the eyes?
    Eyebrows

9. Name a traditional form of repayment or revenge.
    An eye for an eye

10. What piece of material used to cover the eye is often worn by pirates?
    Eye patch

11. To look directly at the eyes of someone is to make what?
    Eye contact

12. What small device is used for administering medications?
    Eyedropper

13. What fringe of hairs grows along the edge of the eyes?
    Eyelashes

14. What portable lens is used to make objects appear larger?
    Eyeglass

15. To make efforts to get someone's attention is to try to do what?
    Catch someone's eye

16. To watch something very closely is to do what?
    Keep your eye on it

17. What is something that is striking, interesting, or attractive called?
    Eye-catching

18. Name an informal exclamation of disagreement.
    My eye!

FACILITATOR: Can the group think of any other phrases or words with an eye in them? Brainstorm other words that have many phrases or objects named after them. You can start with words such as egg, cold, nose, or mind, and then ask the group to think of more. Does everyone agree on the meaning of the expressions or are there a variety of meanings to some of the phrases?

Famous Families

This worksheet lists some of the more well-known families spanning the past century. Based on the information below, try to name the family and some of the more famous members. If you get stumped, choose from the list of families at the bottom of the page for extra help.

1. Which family made its fortune in the shipping and railroad industries during the 19th century?

2. Which family of musicians includes an original member of the Beatles?

3. Which family contains brothers who are famous for their zany comic acts?

4. Which family is famous for its involvement in organized crime?

5. Which famous literary family is responsible for two classic romantic novels?

6. Which American family is famous for its Democratic political involvement?

7. Which family includes theatre and film actors and actresses?

8. Which two families are famous for their decades-long feud?

9. Which family of vocalists has a senior member who was also known as Ol' Blue Eyes?

10. Which family is famous for creating and running the world's largest retailer?

11. Which family made its wealth through the Standard Oil Company and is known for its worldwide philanthropy?

Choices: Barrymore, Sinatra, Lennon, Kennedy, Rockefeller, Marx, Vanderbilt, Gotti, Hatfield, Waltons, Brontë, McCoy

1. Which family made its fortune in the shipping and railroad industries during the 19th century?
    Vanderbilt family—Cornelius, Harold, William Henry

2. Which family of musicians includes an original member of the Beatles?
    Lennon family—John, Julian, Sean, Yoko Ono

3. Which family contains brothers who are famous for their zany comic acts?
    Marx family—Chico, Groucho, Gummo, Harpo, Zeppo

4. Which family is famous for its involvement in organized crime?
    Gotti family—John, Richard, Peter, Victoria

5. Which famous literary family is responsible for two classic romantic novels?
    Brontë family—Anne, Branwell, Charlotte, Emily

6. Which American family is famous for its Democratic political involvement?
    Kennedy family—Caroline, Edward, John, John, Jr., Robert, Rose

7. Which family includes theatre and film actors and actresses?
    Barrymore family—Dolores, Drew, Ethel, John

8. Which two families are famous for their decades-long feud?
    Hatfield and McCoy families—Randolph, William "Devil Anse"

9. Which family of vocalists has a senior member who was also known as Ol' Blue Eyes?
    Sinatra family—Christina, Frank, Frank, Jr., Nancy

10. Which family is famous for creating and running the world's largest retailer?
    Walton family—Helen, Rob, Sam

11. Which family made its wealth through the Standard Oil Company and is known for its worldwide philanthropy?
    Rockefeller family—John, Nelson, William

FACILITATOR: *This is a great exercise for the history buffs in your group. Use this worksheet to encourage people to share their opinions about each of the families. In general, were the families liked or disliked? Respected or looked down on? How do members of each family differ from each other? How are members of your own family alike or different?*

Found in Fours

There are many things that come in, are known by, or are divided into numbers. It often makes it easier for us to remember things this way. The following questions all refer to something that pertains to the number 4. How many items can you identify?

1. What famous foursome made its American debut on *The Ed Sullivan Show* in 1964?

2. What is another name for a homerun?

3. What "good luck" plant has four leaves, rather than the usual three?

4. Name one of the best hands in poker.

5. What is another way to describe 80 years? (*Hint:* Lincoln did it this way.)

6. Spades and hearts are part of what foursome?

7. What divides the year into four parts?

8. What is the name of small, typically French, cakes that are decorated lavishly with frosting?

9. As we get older, sometimes it's hard to get back up when we do what activity?

10. A compass has four what?

11. Many Chevrolets in the 1950s had gears referred to as what?

12. Which four brothers were part of a great family of comedians?

13. What is another name for the clean-up hitter in baseball?

14. What organization for youth focuses on agriculture?

15. The area where Utah, Arizona, New Mexico, and Colorado meet is called what?

16. Sport-utility vans have what feature that allows them to travel in rough terrain?

17. What type of singing group always contains four members who are usually men?

18. Four babies born at one time are called what?

Found in Fours ANSWER SHEET

1. What famous foursome made its American debut on the Ed Sullivan Show in 1964?
   Beatles

2. What is another name for a homerun?
   Four-bagger

3. What "good luck" plant has four leaves, rather than the usual three?
   Four-leaf clover

4. Name one of the best hands in poker.
   Four of a kind

5. What is another way to describe 80 years? (*Hint:* Lincoln did it this way.)
   Four score

6. Spades and hearts are part of what foursome?
   Suits in a deck of cards

7. What divides the year into four parts?
   Seasons

8. What is the name of small, typically French, cakes that are decorated lavishly with frosting?
   Petit fours

9. As we get older, sometimes it's hard to get back up after we do what activity?
   Get down on all fours

10. A compass has four what?
    Directions

11. Many Chevrolets in the 1950s had gears referred to as what?
    Four-on-the-floor

12. Which four brothers were part of a great family of comedians?
    Marx brothers

13. What is another name for the clean-up hitter in baseball?
    Number four batter

14. What organization for youth focuses on agriculture?
    4-H Club

15. The area where Utah, Arizona, New Mexico, and Colorado meet is called what?
    Four corners

16. Sport-utility vans have what feature that allows them to travel in rough terrain?
    4-wheel drive

17. What type of singing group always contains four members who are usually men?
    Barbershop quartet

18. Four babies born at one time are called what?
    Quadruplets

FACILITATOR: *Activities to do with numbers offer a multitude of possibilities for cognitive stimulation. This particular activity focuses on fours, but others could be made up on twos, threes, dozens, and so forth. Follow-up activities could include listing other things pertaining to fours (four horseman, four eyes, four legs on a table, four tires on a car, four-door car, the Four Tops, four quarters in a dollar) and creating a list of things that start with each letter of the alphabet regarding fours (e.g., A—Four Apostles [a famous, controversial painting by Dürer], B—number four batter, C—four leaf clover).*

Games of Childhood

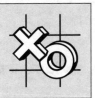

Think back to those after-school, weekend hours, or childhood days of summer when playing was often the first thing on your mind. Match the description on the left with the game on the right.

___ 1. Though many of us did this with one or two ropes to songs or rhymes when we were young, it's used increasingly for fitness.

___ 2. There are many variations to this game, but the basic one has one person being "it" and the rest trying to keep from being touched by "it."

___ 3. This game was first patented in England in 1888 and consists of plastic discs of different colors, a mat, and a container into which the discs are flipped.

___ 4. In this game, you receive $200 for passing "go."

___ 5. "Mary, you may take five big steps" could be one of the instructions given in this game.

___ 6. This game involves a nine-space grid and two opponents, each trying to make a straight line with three of their own markers.

___ 7. This game is played with colorful glass spheres.

___ 8. In this classic game, one person is "it" and the rest try to keep hidden from "it."

___ 9. Played on dark squares, this game requires 12 red pieces and 12 black pieces and is played between two people.

___ 10. In this game, players carefully gather as many sticks as they can without moving the other sticks in the pile.

___ 11. This game involves two teams, each at opposite ends of a rope, pulling as hard as they can.

___ 12. All you need for this game is chalk, a marker for each child, and some "hopping" ability.

___ 13. This game requires a small ball; a hard, level playing surface; and 10 small metal objects.

___ 14. The first person to touch the "stoplight" in this game wins.

___ 15. Everyone must do what the head of the line does in this game.

a. Hide and Seek

b. Follow the Leader

c. Jump rope

d. Tic-Tac-Toe

e. Tug of War

f. Mother, May I?

g. Jacks

h. Tag

i. Checkers

j. Hopscotch

k. Tiddly Winks

l. Pick-Up Sticks

m. Red Light, Green Light

n. Monopoly

o. Marbles

Games of Childhood ANSWER SHEET

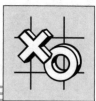

1. Though many of us did this with one or two ropes to songs or rhymes when we were young, it's used increasingly for fitness.

    c. Jump rope

2. There are many variations to this game, but the basic one has one person being "it" and the rest trying to keep from being touched by "it."

    h. Tag

3. This game was first patented in England in 1888 and consists of plastic discs of different colors, a mat, and a container into which the discs are flipped.

    k. Tiddly Winks

4. In this game, you receive $200 for passing "go."

    n. Monopoly

5. "Mary, you may take five big steps" could be one of the instructions given in this game.

    f. Mother, May I?

6. This game involves a nine-space grid and two opponents, each trying to make a straight line with three of their own markers.

    d. Tic-Tac-Toe

7. This game is played with colorful glass spheres.

    o. Marbles

8. In this classic game, one person is "it" and the rest try to keep hidden from "it."

    a. Hide and Seek

9. Played on dark squares, this game requires 12 red pieces and 12 black pieces and is played between two people.

    i. Checkers

10. In this game, players carefully gather as many sticks as they can without moving the other sticks in the pile.

    l. Pick-Up Sticks

11. This game involves two teams, each at opposite ends of a rope, pulling as hard as they can.

    e. Tug of War

12. All you need for this game is chalk, a marker for each child, and some "hopping" ability.

    j. Hopscotch

13. This game requires a small ball; a hard, level playing surface; and 10 small metal objects.

    g. Jacks

14. The first person to touch the "stoplight" in this game wins.

    m. Red Light, Green Light

15. Everyone must do what the head of the line does in this game.

    b. Follow the Leader

FACILITATOR: *This is a great activity for bringing back many childhood memories. As you review the questions, ask participants how many of these games they have played. Which others did they play? With whom? Where? Did they like to play outside or inside best? What was their favorite game? Did they always follow the rules? Did they play any of these games with their children or grandchildren? Do they think that children today "play" as much as they did?*

Gardens and Parks

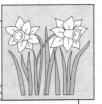

Gardening is one of the most popular pastimes in the United States. Whether you enjoy working in the soil or walking through a flower garden, gardens bring us back to nature's beauty. While you are working on the sheet, use your senses to imagine how each garden would look, what it would smell like, and what the plants would feel like.

___ 1. London is the home to these gardens that cover more than 300 acres and contain a center for botanical research, museums, greenhouses, and the largest plant collection in the world.

___ 2. In this story by Frances Hodgson Burnett, a spoiled orphan finds a key to an abandoned garden and secretly brings the garden back to life.

___ 3. One of the Seven Ancient Wonders of the World, these gardens on the Euphrates River were supposedly built in 600 B.C. by King Nebuchadnezzar II.

___ 4. This famous New York park was the first landscaped public park in the United States and covers 843 acres.

___ 5. The state of New Jersey is known as this.

___ 6. This glass or plastic enclosure is used for growing plants or small animals in a temperature- and humidity-controlled environment.

___ 7. This flower is one of the most popular landscaping shrubs and flowers sold by florists. It is a symbol of love and beauty.

___ 8. This garden is depicted in the book of Genesis as the location where Adam and Eve ate an apple from the Tree of Knowledge.

___ 9. People can try to walk their way through this type of garden that is a maze of paths made out of hedges or plants.

___ 10. This magazine debuted in 1924 to bring articles and information about home décor and gardening.

___ 11. Located in San Francisco, this garden park was once covered in sand dunes but now is more than 1,000 acres and has a variety of attractions, including museums and a herd of bison.

___ 12. Vegetable gardens grow a variety of plants; however, this plant is the most popular to grow for its delicious, sweet bounty.

___ 13. This type of garden has plants clipped or trimmed into neat shapes, sometimes even elaborate animal or person sculptures.

___ 14. Rather than using lots of greenery, this type of garden uses stones for decoration and is also called a rockery or alpine garden.

___ 15. Located in Vancouver, Canada, this 55-acre show garden is more than 100 years old and was built on an old quarry site.

a. Golden Gate Park

b. Kew Gardens

c. Topiary

d. *Better Homes and Gardens*

e. Tomato

f. Central Park

g. *The Secret Garden*

h. Rose

i. Rock garden

j. Garden of Eden

k. Hanging Gardens of Babylon

l. Butchart Gardens

m. Labyrinth

n. Terrarium

o. The Garden State

Gardens and Parks ANSWER SHEET

1. London is the home to these gardens that cover more than 300 acres and contain a center for botanical research, museums, greenhouses, and the largest plant collection in the world.

   b. **Kew Gardens**

2. In this story by Frances Hodgson Burnett, a spoiled orphan finds a key to an abandoned garden and secretly brings the garden back to life.

   g. *The Secret Garden*

3. One of the Seven Ancient Wonders of the World, these gardens on the Euphrates River were supposedly built in 600 B.C. by King Nebuchadnezzar II.

   k. **Hanging Gardens of Babylon**

4. This famous New York park was the first landscaped public park in the United States and covers 843 acres.

   f. **Central Park**

5. The state of New Jersey is known as this.

   o. **The Garden State**

6. This glass or plastic enclosure is used for growing plants or small animals in a temperature- and humidity-controlled environment.

   n. **Terrarium**

7. This flower is one of the most popular landscaping shrubs and flowers sold by florists. It is a symbol of love and beauty.

   h. **Rose**

8. This garden is depicted in the book of Genesis as the location where Adam and Eve ate an apple from the Tree of Knowledge.

   j. **Garden of Eden**

9. People can try to walk their way through this type of garden that is a maze of paths made out of hedges or plants.

   m. **Labyrinth**

10. This magazine debuted in 1924 to bring articles and information about home décor and gardening.

    d. *Better Homes and Gardens*

11. Located in San Francisco, this garden park was once covered in sand dunes but now is more than 1,000 acres and has a variety of attractions, including museums and a herd of bison.

    a. **Golden Gate Park**

12. Vegetable gardens grow a variety of plants; however, this plant is the most popular to grow for its delicious, sweet bounty.

    e. **Tomato**

13. This type of garden has plants clipped or trimmed into neat shapes, sometimes even elaborate animal or person sculptures.

    c. **Topiary**

14. Rather than using lots of greenery, this type of garden uses stones for decoration and is also called a rockery or alpine garden.

    i. **Rock garden**

15. Located in Vancouver, Canada, this 55-acre show garden is more than 100 years old and was built on an old quarry site.

    l. **Butchart Gardens**

FACILITATOR: *Gardens are a wonderful sensory experience. Most of us love gardens. Some of us like to work in them—others would prefer to keep their hands clean! Ask participants who likes gardening. Who likes to visit gardens? What is everyone's favorite flower? Favorite park? Bringing in pictures of some famous parks and gardens, along with some flowers, would add greatly to the sensory pleasure of this activity.*

Strengthen Your Mind by Einberger & Sellick. © 2007 by Health Professions Press, Inc.

Hairstyles of the Decades

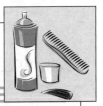

Long or short, blonde, brunette, or redhead, the way we wear our hair says a lot about us. In the past, Hollywood has set precedents for fashionable hairstyles, from the glamorous to the wild. See if you can match the hairstyles described on the left with the answer on the right.

____ 1. This short, neat hairstyle for women was a sign of liberation in the 1920s.

____ 2. This popular 1950s hairstyle featured hair combed back around the sides of the head with the ends sticking out and was popular for young men who wanted to be rebels.

____ 3. This hairstyle became popular in the 1970s and was often seen on hockey players. The hair is worn short on the top and long in the back.

____ 4. This cut, also called the Moe after the Three Stooges character, is worn short on the sides and long and even on the top. It is also called the mushroom cut.

____ 5. With this cut, especially popular with women, hair is worn high and teased on top of the head. The style reached its peak of popularity in the 1960s and is also known as the B-52.

____ 6. This cut is long and neat all around and was made popular in the 1960s by the famous British pop and rock band. It is still enjoyed today.

____ 7. With this style, which is popular with Rastafarians, the hair grows together forming long strands that become thick and matted.

____ 8. In the 1970s, Dorothy Hamill made this look popular. It was created for women but is also worn by men.

____ 9. This cut became synonymous with Punk culture in the 1980s. The hair is shaved on the sides with a strip of hair left on top that can be either short, or long and spiked.

____ 10. This 1950s shoulder-length hairstyle that features the ends curled under is named after a drawing of a woman dressed as an English pageboy.

____ 11. In the 1970s, Farrah Fawcett made this long and layered look popular for young women.

____ 12. This style features hair that is tightly braided in rows along the head.

____ 13. In the 1960s, Mary Tyler Moore made this shoulder length or longer look popular.

____ 14. With this neat look, popular with young girls, the hair is gathered at the top and added in bit by bit, forming a type of braid.

a. French braid

b. Flip

c. Bowl cut

d. Mohawk

e. Dreadlocks

f. Bob

g. Mullet

h. Pageboy

i. Wedge

j. Feathered

k. Cornrows

l. Beatle cut

m. Beehive

n. Ducktail

Hairstyles of the Decades ANSWER SHEET

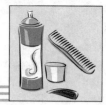

1. This short, neat hairstyle for women was a sign of liberation in the 1920s.

    f.   **Bob**

2. This popular 1950s hairstyle featured hair combed back around the sides of the head with the ends sticking out and was popular for young men who wanted to be rebels.

    n.   **Ducktail**

3. This hairstyle became popular in the 1970s and was often seen on hockey players. The hair is worn short on the top and long in the back.

    g.   **Mullet**

4. This cut, also called the Moe after the Three Stooges character, is worn short on the sides and long and even on the top. It is also called the mushroom cut.

    c.   **Bowl cut**

5. With this cut, especially popular with women, hair is worn high and teased on top of the head. The style reached its peak of popularity in the 1960s and is also known as the B-52.

    m.   **Beehive**

6. This cut is long and neat all around and was made popular in the 1960s by the famous British pop and rock band. It is still enjoyed today.

    l.   **Beatle cut**

7. With this style, which is popular with Rastafarians, the hair grows together forming long strands that become thick and matted.

    e.   **Dreadlocks**

8. In the 1970s, Dorothy Hamill made this look popular. It was created for women but is also worn by men.

    i.   **Wedge**

9. This cut became synonymous with Punk culture in the 1980s. The hair is shaved on the sides with a strip of hair left on top that can be either short, or long and spiked.

    d.   **Mohawk**

10. This 1950s shoulder-length hairstyle that features the ends curled under is named after a drawing of a woman dressed as an English pageboy.

    h.   **Pageboy**

11. In the 1970s, Farrah Fawcett made this long and layered look popular for young women.

    j.   **Feathered**

12. This style features hair that is tightly braided in rows along the head.

    k.   **Cornrows**

13. In the 1960s, Mary Tyler Moore made this shoulder length or longer look popular.

    b.   **Flip**

14. With this neat look, popular with young girls, the hair is gathered at the top and added in bit by bit, forming a type of braid.

    a.   **French braid**

FACILITATOR: *With this worksheet, bring up a discussion about hairstyles that participants have worn. Did anyone wear the above styles? Take a poll of how long it takes each person to "do" his or her hair in the morning. Has anyone ever worn a wig? Where and why? What hairstyles are popular today? How do they differ from those in the past?*

Heroes and Heroines

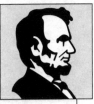

Heroes inspire and impress us; they make the impossible seem possible. Although many of us have our own personal heroes, this worksheet lists a few of the more famous historical and sports figures who may be considered among the greatest heroes of our time. Match the description on the left with the hero or heroine on the right.

_____ 1. This famous boxer's original name was Cassius Clay.

_____ 2. This former president helped to free slaves.

_____ 3. This Catholic nun was known as the "Saint of the Gutters."

_____ 4. This famous golfer is known for bringing the sport to the mainstream in society.

_____ 5. This young girl is famous for her diary that was written while she was in hiding.

_____ 6. This famous baseball player holds the all-time career home run record.

_____ 7. This pilot is famous for his solo flight across the Atlantic Ocean.

_____ 8. This basketball player won six championships and started a Boys and Girls Club in Chicago.

_____ 9. This saint fought the English and was eventually accused of witchcraft and killed.

_____ 10. This runner developed a cult-like following of fans and was killed in an automobile accident at a young age.

_____ 11. This civil rights leader is famous for his "I Have A Dream" speech.

_____ 12. This native of Brazil is considered one of the greatest soccer players of all time.

_____ 13. This individual is famous for being arrested while fighting for women's right to vote.

_____ 14. This person is the first American woman to win three Olympic gold medals.

_____ 15. This Mexican-American activist's campaigning led to major improvements for farm workers.

a. Michael Jordan

b. Hank Aaron

c. Abraham Lincoln

d. Pelé

e. Joan of Arc

f. César Chávez

g. Arnold Palmer

h. Anne Frank

i. Muhammad Ali

j. Mother Teresa

k. Wilma Rudolph

l. Susan B. Anthony

m. Steve Prefontaine

n. Charles Lindbergh

o. Martin Luther King, Jr.

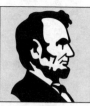

Heroes and Heroines ANSWER SHEET

1. This famous boxer's original name was Cassius Clay.   **i.   Muhammad Ali**

2. This former president helped to free slaves.   **c.   Abraham Lincoln**

3. This Catholic nun was known as the "Saint of the Gutters."   **j.   Mother Teresa**

4. This famous golfer is known for bringing the sport to the
   mainstream in society.   **g.   Arnold Palmer**

5. This young girl is famous for her diary that was written
   while she was in hiding.   **h.   Anne Frank**

6. This famous baseball player holds the all-time career
   home run record.   **b.   Hank Aaron**

7. This pilot is famous for his solo flight across the Atlantic
   Ocean.   **n.   Charles Lindbergh**

8. This basketball player won six championships and started
   a Boys and Girls Club in Chicago.   **a.   Michael Jordan**

9. This saint fought the English and was eventually accused
   of witchcraft and killed.   **e.   Joan of Arc**

10. This runner developed a cult-like following of fans and
    was killed in an automobile accident at a young age.   **m.   Steve Prefontaine**

11. This civil rights leader is famous for his "I Have A Dream"
    speech.   **o.   Martin Luther King, Jr.**

12. This native of Brazil is considered one of the greatest
    soccer players of all time.   **d.   Pelé**

13. This individual is famous for being arrested while fighting
    for women's right to vote.   **l.   Susan B. Anthony**

14. This person is the first American woman to win three
    Olympic gold medals.   **k.   Wilma Rudolph**

15. This Mexican-American activist's campaigning led to
    major improvements for farm workers.   **f.   César Chávez**

FACILITATOR: *After participants have completed all they can, encourage conversation about individual heroes. Who are their personal heroes? Who else would they add or remove from this list? What else do they know about each of the people listed here?*

Strengthen Your Mind by Einberger & Sellick. © 2007 by Health Professions Press, Inc.

I Scream, You Scream . . .

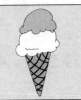

One of America's most popular desserts, ice cream comes in dozens of flavors. From store bought to homemade, ice cream is a sweet treat that people of all ages enjoy. For a fun (and appetizing) mental workout, answer the questions below.

1. Name the three basic ingredients that give ice cream its delicious, creamy flavor.

2. Which type of ice cream is really not creamy at all? (*Hint:* It is based with water, giving it a lighter taste.)

3. List at least three ice cream flavors that contain nuts.

4. Which decadent dessert is made with a banana, three ice cream flavors, toppings, and whipped cream?

5. With which flavor of ice cream do you get three flavors in one: chocolate, vanilla, and strawberry?

6. Which popular alternative to ice cream is made from another source of dairy and is generally lower in fat?

7. List at least three brands of ice cream that are commonly found at most grocery stores.

8. Which edible device for holding ice cream was originally made from glass or metal (called a *penny lick*) or wrapped paper (called a *hokey pokey)?*

9. Although everyone has his or her favorite, which flavor of ice cream is America's most popular?

10. Baskin-Robbins, the world's largest ice cream franchise, is famous for having how many flavors?

11. Before the invention of electric ice cream makers, if you wanted to make ice cream at home you had to use what?

12. Beware of eating ice cream too fast. If you do, you may suffer from what?

13. What Italian ice cream is typically made with chocolate and pistachio flavors and contains fruit and nuts?

14. Which flavor of ice cream is a blend of chocolate ice cream mixed with marshmallow and almonds?

I Scream, You Scream . . . ANSWER SHEET

1. Name the three basic ingredients that give ice cream its delicious, creamy flavor.
   Cream, milk, sugar

2. Which type of ice cream is really not creamy at all? (*Hint:* It is based with water, giving it a lighter taste.)
   Ice milk

3. List at least three ice cream flavors that contain nuts.
   Black walnut, butter pecan, pecan praline, pistachio, rocky road

4. Which decadent dessert is made with a banana, three ice cream flavors, toppings, and whipped cream?
   Banana split

5. With which flavor of ice cream do you get three flavors in one: chocolate, vanilla, and strawberry?
   Neapolitan

6. Which popular alternative to ice cream is made from another source of dairy and is generally lower in fat?
   Frozen yogurt

7. List at least three brands of ice cream that are commonly found at most grocery stores.
   Ben & Jerry's, Breyers, Dreyer's, Häagen-Dazs

8. Which edible device for holding ice cream was originally made from glass or metal (called a *penny lick)* or wrapped paper (called a *hokey pokey)*?
   Ice cream cone

9. Although everyone has his or her favorite, which flavor of ice cream is America's most popular?
   Vanilla

10. Baskin-Robbins, the world's largest ice cream franchise, is famous for having how many flavors?
    Thirty-one

11. Before the invention of electric ice cream makers, if you wanted to make ice cream at home you had to use what?
    Hand crank

12. Beware of eating ice cream too fast. If you do, you may suffer from what?
    Brain freeze or ice cream headache

13. What Italian ice cream is typically made with chocolate and pistachio flavors and contains fruit and nuts?
    Spumoni

14. Which flavor of ice cream is a blend of chocolate ice cream mixed with marshmallow and almonds?
    Rocky road

FACILITATOR: *The topic of ice cream is bound to bring up a variety of discussions. What is everyone's favorite flavor? Least favorite flavor? Is there anyone who doesn't like ice cream? If participants could create their own flavor, what would it be? Make an A-to-Z list of ice cream flavors. If you can, have a few different flavors of ice cream to taste, and encourage participants to use their senses to really enjoy the treat.*

80   *Strengthen Your Mind* by Einberger & Sellick. © 2007 by Health Professions Press, Inc.

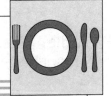

Indian, Italian, French, and Other Regional Foods

More and more, ethnic foods are found in stores, in restaurants, at the dinner tables of friends. "American" food is expanding! Each of the following foods is particularly associated with a state, area or foreign country. Can you name these places?

1. Yorkshire pudding (popover-like bread served with roast beef)

2. Gelato (dense, rich ice cream)

3. Hummus (mixture containing mashed chickpeas)

4. Ratatouille (vegetable stew)

5. Poi (fermented paste made from taro root)

6. Sushi (raw fish and rice, wrapped in seaweed)

7. Chai (sweet, spiced tea)

8. Paella (rice dish with meat, seafood, and vegetables)

9. Chianti (dry, red wine)

10. Crepes (thin pancakes)

11. Sauerbraten (marinated beef cooked with vinegar)

12. Baklava (sweet pastry of phyllo dough, nuts, spice, and honey-lemon syrup)

13. Escargots (edible snails)

14. Chutney (relish made from fruit, spices, and herbs)

15. Grits (coarsely ground corn)

16. Goulash (stew seasoned with paprika)

17. Tamales (meat filling wrapped in cornhusks)

18. Tapas (small appetizers)

19. Schnitzel (fried veal cutlet)

20. Sake (wine made from rice)

Indian, Italian, French, and Other Regional Foods
ANSWER SHEET

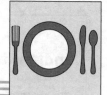

1.	Yorkshire pudding	**England**
2.	Gelato	**Italy**
3.	Hummus	**Middle East**
4.	Ratatouille	**France**
5.	Poi	**Hawaii**
6.	Sushi	**Japan**
7.	Chai	**India**
8.	Paella	**Spain**
9.	Chianti	**Italy**
10.	Crepes	**France**
11.	Sauerbraten	**Germany**
12.	Baklava	**Greece/Turkey**
13.	Escargots	**France**
14.	Chutney	**India**
15.	Grits	**Southern United States**
16.	Goulash	**Hungary**
17.	Tamales	**Mexico**
18.	Tapas	**Spain**
19.	Schnitzel	**Austria**
20.	Sake	**Japan**

FACILITATOR: *Ethnic foods are becoming more and more popular throughout the United States and the world. Discuss with participants other specialties from these countries. Which ones have they eaten? What are their favorites? Have they ever prepared these dishes? Which ethnicity of food do they like best? Do they have favorite ethnic restaurants? What do they order?*

Jiminy Cricket and Other Fictional Characters

Over the past century, fictional characters from radio, movie, print, and television have delighted and entertained us. Although the characters below are just a few of the many, they are some of the more famous personalities from a variety of media. Read each question, and name the fictional character to which it refers.

1. Which British outlaw lived in Sherwood Forest and robbed from the rich to feed the poor?

2. What famous lumberjack did his work with his faithful blue ox, Babe, and his seven axmen, all named Elmer?

3. What "man of steel" is known for being "faster than a speeding bullet" and is the most popular comic book character of all time?

4. Which cheery character first appeared in 1928 and is known worldwide as the symbol of Disneyland, the happiest place on earth?

5. Which British mythological figure became the leader of the Knights of the Roundtable?

6. Which detective solved mysteries from his home at 221B Baker Street with the help of his dear friend, Dr. Watson?

7. Gene Wilder portrayed which character in the 1971 film where a boy wins the "golden ticket" and gets to tour a magical chocolate factory?

8. Which character, who lives among the apes in the jungle and swings from the vines, made his first appearance in 1912?

9. What fictional British spy, known as "007," has a reputation for being a womanizer and was first portrayed by Sean Connery?

10. What bald-headed character was Little Orphan Annie's adoptive father in the 1924 comic strip and in later productions of the story?

11. What pet beagle is Charlie Brown's friend and is known for sleeping on his doghouse and enjoying the company of his good friend, Woodstock?

12. What vain and selfish character in the movie *Gone with the Wind* was torn between her love for a southern gentleman, Ashley, and a smooth ladies man, Rhett?

13. Which leading character in *The Maltese Falcon* was famously portrayed by Humphrey Bogart?

14. What ill-tempered, frugal man gets a visit from the ghosts of Christmas past, present, and future in *A Christmas Carol* by Charles Dickens?

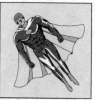

Jiminy Cricket and Other Fictional Characters
ANSWER SHEET

1. Which British outlaw lived in Sherwood Forest and robbed from the rich to feed the poor?
   Robin Hood

2. What famous lumberjack did his work with his faithful blue ox, Babe and his seven axmen, all named Elmer?
   Paul Bunyan

3. What "man of steel" is known for being "faster than a speeding bullet" and is the most popular comic book character of all time?
   Superman

4. Which cheery character first appeared in 1928 and is known worldwide as the symbol of Disneyland, the happiest place on earth?
   Mickey Mouse

5. Which British mythological figure became the leader of the Knights of the Roundtable?
   King Arthur

6. Which detective solved mysteries from his home at 221B Baker Street with the help of his dear friend, Dr. Watson?
   Sherlock Holmes

7. Gene Wilder portrayed which character in the 1971 film where a boy wins a "golden ticket" and gets to tour a magical chocolate factory?
   Willy Wonka

8. Which character, who lives among the apes in the jungle and swings from the vines, made his first appearance in 1912?
   Tarzan

9. What fictional British spy, known as "007," has a reputation for being a womanizer and was first portrayed by Sean Connery?
   James Bond

10. What bald-headed character was Little Orphan Annie's adoptive father in the 1924 comic strip and in later productions of the story?
    Daddy Warbucks

11. What pet beagle is Charlie Brown's friend and is known for sleeping on his doghouse and enjoying the company of his good friend, Woodstock?
    Snoopy

12. What vain and selfish character in the movie *Gone with the Wind* was torn between her love for a southern gentleman, Ashley, and a smooth ladies man, Rhett?
    Scarlett O'Hara

13. Which leading character in *The Maltese Falcon* was famously portrayed by Humphrey Bogart?
    Sam Spade

14. What ill-tempered, frugal man gets a visit from the ghosts of Christmas past, present, and future in *A Christmas Carol* by Charles Dickens?
    Ebenezer Scrooge

FACILITATOR: *Fictional characters have added to our enjoyment of movies, books, television shows, and more for many, many years. Ask participants for their favorites. Who are other fictional characters? Which current favorites do they recognize? Shrek? The Little Mermaid?*

   Strengthen Your Mind by Einberger & Sellick. © 2007 by Health Professions Press, Inc.

Joie de Vivre = Enjoyment of Life
Common Foreign Words and Phrases

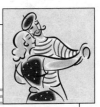

English-speakers use words from foreign languages routinely in their everyday lives. The following commonly used words and expressions are all derived from different languages. Give the meaning of each word or phrase, and, for extra "bonus" points, name the language of origin. The dictionary may be helpful with some of these!

Word or phrase	Meaning	Language of origin
1. Bonjour		
2. C'est la vie		
3. Modus operandi		
4. Buenos días		
5. Cosa Nostra		
6. La dolce vita		
7. Faux pas		
8. Tête-à-tête		
9. Mea culpa		
10. Persona non grata		
11. Double-entendre		
12. Carte blanche		
13. Verboten		
14. Alfresco		
15. Savoir-faire		
16. Veni, vidi, vici		
17. Voilà		
18. Adiós		
19. Merci		
20. Crème de la crème		

Joie de Vivre = Enjoyment of Life
Common Foreign Words and Phrases ANSWER SHEET

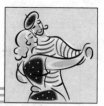

Word or phrase	Meaning	Language of origin
1. Bonjour	Hello	French
2. C'est la vie	That's life	French
3. Modus operandi	Method of operating	Latin
4. Buenos días	Good day	Spanish
5. Cosa Nostra	Mafia	Italian
6. La dolce vita	The good life	Italian
7. Faux pas	A social blunder	French
8. Tête-à-tête	A close chat	French
9. Mea culpa	I am to blame	Latin
10. Persona non grata	Unacceptable or unwelcome person	Latin
11. Double-entendre	Having two different meanings	French
12. Carte blanche	Unrestricted power to act on one's own	French
13. Verboten	Forbidden	German
14. Alfresco	In the open air, outside	Italian
15. Savoir-faire	Knowing how to act appropriately	French
16. Veni, vidi, vici	I came, I saw, I conquered	Latin
17. Voilà	Behold	French
18. Adiós	Good-bye	Spanish
19. Merci	Thank you	French
20. Crème de la crème	The very best	French

FACILITATOR: After participants have completed as much as they can, ask the following questions: Who speaks a foreign language? Who knows other common words in foreign languages? Where do most of our words come from? Do you think that other languages use English words, too, and, if so, which ones? Try introducing a foreign word into an activity occasionally.

Keys to Everything

Did you know that many phrases and items are associated with the word *key*? The answers to the questions below all have the word *key* in them (except #16). Use your creativity to come up with the answers, and ask friends or family if you need extra help.

1. What chain of islands is located along the Caribbean Sea and is more than 100 miles long?

2. What keys are black and white and can make a beautiful sound when pressed?

3. What slightly sour pie is a cool, refreshing treat for dessert?

4. A person who begins a conference or other large gathering delivers what type of presentation?

5. A vocalist whose voice sounds pleasant can be thought to sing in what way?

6. Too many keys can be a nuisance. Many people carry their keys on what?

7. What club can high school students join that promotes leadership through service?

8. Who wrote the *The Star Spangled Banner,* which officially became our national anthem on March 3, 1931?

9. With what type of key can you open several doors?

10. What machine, which resembled a small desk, was used to manually enter data onto a punch card?

11. In the early 1900s, which policemen were famous for their funny but silent antics on film?

12. What machine resembles a piano but is portable and can be used with battery power?

13. What is pressing a key on a keyboard called?

14. What popular keychain symbolizes good luck and is made from the "foot" of a certain animal?

15. Which city in Florida is the southernmost city in the continental United States and was home to Ernest Hemingway for more than 10 years?

16. The "keys" in basketball are located on which part of the court?

Keys to Everything ANSWER SHEET

1. What chain of islands is located along the Caribbean Sea and is more than 100 miles long?
    Florida Keys

2. What keys are black and white and can make a beautiful sound when pressed?
    Piano keys

3. What slightly sour pie is a cool, refreshing treat for dessert?
    Key lime pie

4. A person who begins a conference or other large gathering delivers what type of presentation?
    Keynote address, presentation, or speech

5. A vocalist whose voice sounds pleasant can be thought to sing in what way?
    In key

6. Too many keys can be a nuisance. Many people carry their keys on what?
    Keychain

7. What club can high school students join that promotes leadership through service?
    Key Club

8. Who wrote *The Star Spangled Banner*, which officially became our national anthem on March 3, 1931?
    Francis Scott Key

9. With what type of key can you open several doors?
    Master key, passkey, or skeleton key

10. What machine, which resembled a small desk, was used to manually enter data onto a punch card?
    Keypunch

11. In the early 1900s, which policemen were famous for their funny but silent antics on film?
    Keystone Cops

12. What machine resembles a piano but is portable and can be used with battery power?
    Keyboard

13. What is pressing a key on a keyboard called?
    Keystroke

14. What popular keychain symbolizes good luck and is made from the "foot" of a certain animal?
    Rabbit foot keychain

15. Which city in Florida is the southernmost city in the continental United States and was home to Ernest Hemingway for more than 10 years?
    Key West, Florida

16. The "keys" in basketball are located on which part of the court?
    At each end of the court

FACILITATOR: *This is just a partial list of words associated with the word key. Ask participants if they can name any others. For further conversation, encourage discussion about the different keys that people have carried in their lifetime. Ask participants the following questions: When did you get keys to your first car? First house? Keys to your office or workplace? How did it feel to call them your own? Did you ever carry a keychain that held special meaning?*

Strengthen Your Mind by Einberger & Sellick. © 2007 by Health Professions Press, Inc.

Kiss a Toad and Other Superstitions

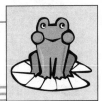

Whether you believe in them or not, superstitions—good and bad—are related to many aspects of our daily lives. Below is a list of items that are the basis of common superstitions. Read the item and list as many superstitions as you can think of that are related to each item.

1. Apple

2. Ladder

3. Cat

4. Bell

5. Umbrella

6. Mirror

7. Clover

8. Horseshoe

9. Salt

10. Ears

11. Dandelion

12. Star

13. Flag

14. Door

15. Baseball bat

16. Birthday cake

17. Eyelash

18. Friday the 13th

19. Wishbone

20. Blarney Stone

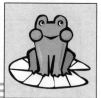

1. Apple — An apple a day keeps the doctor away.

   Twist the stem of an apple while saying the letters of the alphabet. Whichever letter the stem falls off on is the first letter of the name of the person that you will marry.

2. Ladder — It is bad luck to walk under a ladder.

3. Cat — A black cat on a ship is bad luck.

   If a black cat walks toward you, it brings good luck. If it walks away again, it takes the good luck with it.

4. Bell — Every time a bell rings, an angel gets its wings.

5. Umbrella — It is bad luck to open an umbrella in the house.

6. Mirror — To break a mirror means 7 years of bad luck.

7. Clover — A person who keeps a four-leaf clover in the house is protected from spells.

   To find a four-leaf clover is good luck.

8. Horseshoe — Hang a horseshoe above a doorway to bring good luck to the house.

9. Salt — If you spill salt, you will have bad luck unless you throw a pinch over your shoulder.

10. Ears — If your ears itch, it means someone is talking ill of you.

11. Dandelion — If you blow on a dandelion gone to seed and make a wish, the wish will come true.

    The number of seeds left on a dandelion after you blow on it is the number of children you will have.

12. Star — Make a wish on a shooting star, and it will come true.

13. Flag — It is bad luck for a flag to touch the ground.

14. Door — It is bad luck to leave through a different door than you came in through.

15. Baseball bat — Spit on a baseball bat to make it lucky.

16. Birthday cake — Make a wish when you blow out birthday candles, and it will come true.

17. Eyelash — If an eyelash falls out, put it on the back of your hand, and blow it over your shoulder. If it flies off your hand, your wish will be granted.

18. Friday the 13th — Friday the 13th is a day of bad luck.

    Friday is considered the most unlucky day of the week, and the number 13 has historical and biblical references to bad luck.

19. Wishbone — When two people pull on opposite sides of a dry wishbone, the person who ends up with the bigger side will have his or her wish come true.

20. Blarney Stone — If you kiss the Blarney Stone (set in Blarney Castle, Ireland), you will be given the gift of blarney (persuasive eloquence).

FACILITATOR: Encourage participants to brainstorm all of the superstitions and beliefs that they have about the items above. Ask participants if there is any truth to the above superstitions. What are some other old wives tales that are not listed above?

Lakes, Rivers, and Other Bodies of Water

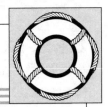

Much of our lives are centered around waterways—the rivers we fish in, the creeks we jump over, the lakes we swim in, and the oceans we sail in or fly over. Many of these bodies of water are well known. The following ones are located throughout the world. Can you name them?

1. What is the largest freshwater lake in the world?

2. Europeans flock to the coast of which sea in the summer?

3. What is the biggest bay in the world?

4. What is the longest river in the world?

5. What New Mexican river is home to many western movies?

6. What is the largest ocean?

7. How much of the earth's surface is covered with water? (*Hint:* Is it 25%, 50%, or 70%?)

8. What river runs through the Grand Canyon?

9. What river does the jungle keep almost hidden for hundreds of miles in South America?

10. On what river are Big Ben and the Houses of Parliament located?

11. Lewis and Clark finished their journey at the mouth of what river?

12. On what river did Tom Sawyer and Huck Finn have their rafting adventures?

13. Name the five oceans.

14. Notre Dame in Paris is located on which river?

15. Which river, Europe's second largest, is often described as very blue and has a Strauss waltz named after it?

16. What 51-mile–long waterway connects the Pacific and the Atlantic Oceans in Central America?

17. What type of waterway, formed by glaciers, are Norway and Alaska both well known for having?

Lakes, Rivers, and Other Bodies of Water
ANSWER SHEET

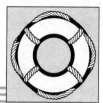

1. What is the largest freshwater lake in the world?
   Lake Superior

2. Europeans flock to the coast of which sea in the summer?
   Mediterranean Sea

3. What is the biggest bay in the world?
   Hudson Bay

4. What is the longest river in the world?
   Nile River

5. What New Mexican river is home to many western movies?
   Rio Grande

6. What is the largest ocean?
   Pacific Ocean

7. How much of the earth's surface is covered with water? (*Hint:* Is it 25%, 50%, or 70%?)
   70%

8. What river runs through the Grand Canyon?
   Colorado River

9. What river does the jungle keep almost hidden for hundreds of miles in South America?
   Amazon River

10. On what river are Big Ben and the Houses of Parliament located?
    Thames River

11. Lewis and Clark finished their journey at the mouth of what river?
    Columbia River

12. On what river did Tom Sawyer and Huck Finn have their rafting adventures?
    Mississippi River

13. Name the five oceans.
    Antarctic Ocean, Arctic Ocean, Atlantic Ocean, Indian Ocean, Pacific Ocean

14. Notre Dame in Paris is located on which river?
    Seine River

15. Which river, Europe's second longest, is often described as very blue and has a Strauss waltz named after it?
    Danube River

16. What 51-mile–long waterway connects the Pacific and the Atlantic Oceans in Central America?
    Panama Canal

17. What type of waterway, formed by glaciers, are Norway and Alaska both well known for having?
    Fjords (or fiords)

FACILITATOR: *As noted above, 70% of the earth is covered in water. These thousands of bodies of water offer many topics of discussion. How many lakes, rivers, seas, and so forth can participants name? Which ones have they visited? Would they like to live on a lake or a river? Have they been involved in water sports—swimming, skiing, fishing? What historical events have taken place on water? As with all of the activity sheets that involve geography, be sure to use a map.*

Strengthen Your Mind by Einberger & Sellick. © 2007 by Health Professions Press, Inc.

License Plates of the United States

Automobile license plates are used throughout the world to identify to whom the vehicle is registered and where it is registered. In addition to identification purposes, license plates have also been the focus of travel games. One such game was trying to find plates from each of the 50 states in the shortest time possible. Often this took hours! Identify which state uses or used the following slogans on their license plates.

1. The First State

2. The Last Frontier

3. Land of Enchantment

4. The Silver State

5. Garden State

6. Grand Canyon State

7. Big Sky

8. Famous Potatoes

9. Show-Me State

10. Land of Lincoln

11. 10,000 Lakes

12. World's Motor Capital

13. Great Faces, Great Places

14. Volunteer State

15. Greatest Snow on Earth

16. Green Mountain State

17. The Empire State

18. Sunshine State

License Plates of the United States ANSWER SHEET

1. The First State   **Delaware**

2. The Last Frontier   **Alaska**

3. Land of Enchantment   **New Mexico**

4. The Silver State   **Nevada**

5. Garden State   **New Jersey**

6. Grand Canyon State   **Arizona**

7. Big Sky   **Montana**

8. Famous Potatoes   **Idaho**

9. Show-Me State   **Missouri**

10. Land of Lincoln   **Illinois**

11. 10,000 Lakes   **Minnesota**

12. World's Motor Capital   **Michigan**

13. Great Faces, Great Places   **South Dakota**

14. Volunteer State   **Tennessee**

15. Greatest Snow on Earth   **Utah**

16. Green Mountain State   **Vermont**

17. The Empire State   **New York**

18. Sunshine State   **Florida**

FACILITATOR: *Chances are, many participants were born in the above states and are well aware of the license plates. Ask for the meaning of the descriptions. Do they know those of other states? Do they remember the color of their license plate? Have the colors changed over the years? Did they play games using license plates when they were young? When they were raising children? Which license plates were most difficult to find? How many states have they been to? Do they save license plates or did they do so in the past? Using a map would be helpful.*

Strengthen Your Mind by Einberger & Sellick. © 2007 by Health Professions Press, Inc.

Measurements

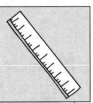

Our everyday lives are filled with measurements—how much apples weigh at the grocery store, how much flour we put in the cookies, how far we've walked. We measure things in many different ways—on a scale, in a measuring cup, on a thermometer, and much more. Think about these different ways as you try to identify the following measurements.

1. There are 4 cups in a what?

2. What unit are horses measured in?

3. How many items are in a baker's dozen?

4. How many time zones are there in the world?

5. There are 3 teaspoons in a what?

6. What is a counting device with a frame and rods with moveable beads called?

7. There are 4 pecks in a what?

8. There are 2 cups in a what?

9. One decade equals how many years?

10. What unit of length is used in ship navigation?

11. Mph stands for what?

12. There are 4 quarts in a what?

13. How many days are in a leap year?

14. How many degrees are in a circle?

15. How many fluid ounces are in 1 cup?

16. How many inches are in 1 foot?

17. How many yards are there in a football field?

18. What is the average body temperature for most people?

1. There are 4 cups in a what?
   Quart

2. What unit are horses measured in?
   Hands

3. How many items are in a baker's dozen?
   13

4. How many time zones are there in the world?
   24

5. There are 3 teaspoons in a what?
   Tablespoon

6. What is a counting device with a frame and rods with moveable beads called?
   Abacus

7. There are 4 pecks in a what?
   Bushel

8. There are 2 cups in a what?
   Pint

9. One decade equals how many years?
   10

10. What unit of length is used in ship navigation?
    Nautical mile

11. Mph stands for what?
    Miles per hour

12. There are 4 quarts in a what?
    Gallon

13. How many days are in a leap year?
    366

14. How many degrees are in a circle?
    360

15. How many fluid ounces are in 1 cup?
    8

16. How many inches are in 1 foot?
    12

17. How many yards are there in a football field?
    100

18. What is the average body temperature for most people?
    98.6° F

FACILITATOR: When reviewing this sheet, it would be good to have out items used for measuring, such as a ruler, a measuring cup, a thermometer, and a calendar. Ask for other tools used for measuring. Ask participants the following questions: What else do we measure on a regular basis? Did you use a slide rule, a protractor, a compass, a calculator, or an adding machine? Are children today losing the ability to do math in their heads? Is math made too easy with calculators?

Mountains and Deserts of the World

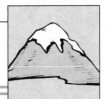

Mountains cover about one fifth of the earth's surface. Deserts cover approximately another fifth. From the lowest elevations in the world to the highest, many have become famous for a variety of reasons. Match the facts on the left with the mountain(s) and deserts on the right that they describe.

_____ 1. This is the highest peak in the world.

_____ 2. This western U.S. mountain range is home to many volcanoes, including Mt. St. Helens.

_____ 3. This mountain range, the longest in the world, is located along the western coast of South America.

_____ 4. In 1980, this volcano in Washington erupted for the first time in 120 years.

_____ 5. Europeans flock to world-class ski resorts in these mountains in the heart of Switzerland.

_____ 6. This is the only continent that does not contain deserts.

_____ 7. These mountains are home to the tallest peaks in the world.

_____ 8. These mountains separate France and Spain.

_____ 9. These mountains are home to the Pennsylvania Dutch.

_____ 10. These mountains are so named because of the bluish haze surrounding them.

_____ 11. This mountain range runs from northwest Alaska to the Mexican border.

_____ 12. This is the largest nonpolar desert in the world.

_____ 13. This mountain erupted in A.D. 79, burying Pompeii.

_____ 14. This sacred mountain is the highest in Japan.

_____ 15. The California Gold Rush took place in the foothills of these mountains.

_____ 16. This desert is located in Southern California, Utah, Nevada, and Arizona.

a. Great Smokies

b. Appalachians

c. Sahara Desert

d. Sierra Nevadas

e. Mt. Vesuvius

f. Cascades

g. Pyrenees

h. Mt. Everest

i. Alps

j. Rockies

k. Andes

l. Mojave Desert

m. Mt. St. Helens

n. Europe

o. Himalayas

p. Mt. Fuji

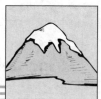

Mountains and Deserts of the World ANSWER SHEET

1. This is the highest peak in the world.   **h.   Mt. Everest**

2. This western U.S. mountain range is home to many   **f.   Cascades**
   volcanoes, including Mt. St. Helens.

3. This mountain range, the longest in the world, is   **k.   Andes**
   located along the western coast of South America.

4. In 1980, this volcano in Washington erupted for the   **m. Mt. St. Helens**
   first time in 120 years.

5. Europeans flock to world-class ski resorts in these   **i.   Alps**
   mountains in the heart of Switzerland.

6. This is the only continent that does not contain   **n.   Europe**
   deserts.

7. These mountains are home to the tallest peaks in   **o.   Himalayas**
   the world.

8. These mountains separate France and Spain.   **g.   Pyrenees**

9. These mountains are home to the Pennsylvania   **b.   Appalachians**
   Dutch.

10. These mountains are so named because of the bluish   **a.   Great Smokies**
    haze surrounding them.

11. This mountain range runs from northwest Alaska to the   **j.   Rockies**
    Mexican border.

12. This is the largest nonpolar desert in the world.   **c.   Sahara Desert**

13. This mountain erupted in A.D. 79, burying Pompeii.   **e.   Mt. Vesuvius**

14. This sacred mountain is the highest in Japan.   **p.   Mt. Fuji**

15. The California Gold Rush took place in the foothills of   **d.   Sierra Nevadas**
    these mountains.

16. This desert is located in Southern California, Utah,   **l.   Mojave Desert**
    Nevada, and Arizona.

FACILITATOR: *Most participants have visited at least one of these mountains, mountain ranges, or deserts. Start by asking which ones each person has visited. Follow-up questions may include: Would you like to visit these places? Would you like to climb these mountains? Would you rather live in the mountains or on the beach? Is there any particular history associated with these places? Can you name other major deserts and mountain ranges? Be sure to use a map when discussing this activity.*

Strengthen Your Mind by Einberger & Sellick. © 2007 by Health Professions Press, Inc.

National Parks and Other U.S. Landmarks

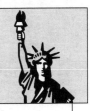

The United States is full of wonderful attractions, some natural and others manmade. Most of us need only travel a short distance to see one or more of these attractions. Take a trip around the United States and identify the following attractions.

1. Which California National Park is home to the highest waterfall in the United States (2,425 feet—the fifth largest in the world)?

2. Which stone monument, located in South Dakota, is a tribute to four very important people?

3. Which is the most visited (9 million annually) national park?

4. Which California park is home to the world's tallest trees?

5. Which New York building was the tallest skyscraper in the world for 41 years?

6. What is the world's greatest geyser area (and also the oldest national park—1872)?

7. Which park was the site of the largest battle of the Civil War?

8. Two hundred seventy-seven miles of the Colorado River run through which park in Arizona?

9. The site of the lowest elevation in the Western Hemisphere—282 feet below sea level—is called what?

10. Which New York monument is a symbol of freedom and democracy?

11. Which New Orleans area is home to the famous Mardi Gras celebration?

12. Main Street U.S.A. serves as the entrance to which famous theme park?

13. What water attraction, which straddles the U.S.–Canadian border, attracts approximately 12 million tourists each year?

14. Which mountain, named *Denali,* or "the high one," by Native Americans, has the highest peak in the United States?

15. Which attraction opened in 1962 and was the focus of the World's Fair in Seattle?

National Parks and Other U.S. Landmarks ANSWER SHEET

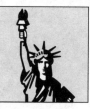

1. Which California National Park is home to the highest waterfall in the United States (2,425 feet—the fifth largest in the world)?
   Yosemite National Park

2. Which stone monument, located in South Dakota, is a tribute to four very important people?
   Mt. Rushmore National Memorial

3. Which is the most visited (9 million annually) national park?
   Great Smoky Mountains National Park

4. Which California park is home to the world's tallest trees?
   Redwood National Park

5. Which New York building was the tallest skyscraper in the world for 41 years?
   Empire State Building

6. What is the world's greatest geyser area (and also the oldest national park—1872)?
   Yellowstone National Park

7. Which park is the site of the largest battle of the Civil War?
   Gettysburg National Military Park

8. Two hundred seventy-seven miles of the Colorado River run through which park in Arizona?
   Grand Canyon National Park

9. The site of the lowest elevation in the Western Hemisphere—282 feet below sea level— is called what?
   Death Valley

10. Which New York monument is a symbol of freedom and democracy?
    Statue of Liberty

11. Which New Orleans area is home to the famous Mardi Gras celebration?
    Bourbon Street or the French Quarter

12. Main Street U.S.A. serves as the entrance to which famous theme park?
    Disneyland or Walt Disney World

13. What water attraction, which straddles the U.S.–Canadian border, attracts approximately 12 million tourists each year?
    Niagara Falls

14. Which mountain, named *Denali,* or "the high one," by Native Americans, has the highest peak in the United States?
    Mt. McKinley

15. Which attraction opened in 1962 and was the focus of the World's Fair in Seattle?
    Space Needle

FACILITATOR: *Most participants have visited at least one of our nation's parks or manmade attractions. Discuss who has been to which park. Ask participants which parks they think are most popular and why. What makes a place suitable to be named a national park? Are there places that participants think should be national parks but are not? It's important to have a map as a visual aid when discussing the answers to this activity. After discussing parks, ask many of the same questions regarding our nation's manmade tourist attractions. Which would participants rather visit—a natural or a manmade attraction?*

Strengthen Your Mind by Einberger & Sellick. © 2007 by Health Professions Press, Inc.

Nicknames of the Famous and Infamous

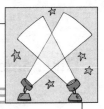

Nicknames have been used throughout history to describe people, places, and so forth. These nicknames can refer to physical characteristics, occupations, personalities, nationalities, backgrounds, special feats, and more. Identify the following people based on their nicknames.

1. The Georgia Peach

2. Leader of the Rough Riders

3. The Girl with the Curls

4. The Brown Bomber

5. The King of Late Night Television

6. The Peanut Farmer

7. The Bard of Avon

8. Satchmo

9. The Sultan of Swat

10. The "It" Girl

11. The Rail Splitter

12. The Lone Eagle

13. Buffalo Bill

14. Il Duce

15. The Duke

16. Scarface

17. The Desert Fox

18. Ol' Blue Eyes

19. Superman

20. Schnozzola

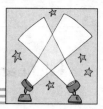

1. The Georgia Peach — **Ty Cobb**

2. Leader of the Rough Riders — **Theodore Roosevelt**

3. The Girl with the Curls — **Shirley Temple**

4. The Brown Bomber — **Joe Louis**

5. The King of Late Night Television — **Johnny Carson**

6. The Peanut Farmer — **Jimmy Carter**

7. The Bard of Avon — **William Shakespeare**

8. Satchmo — **Louis Armstrong**

9. The Sultan of Swat — **Babe Ruth**

10. The "It" Girl — **Clara Bow**

11. The Rail Splitter — **Abraham Lincoln**

12. The Lone Eagle — **Charles Lindbergh**

13. Buffalo Bill — **William Cody**

14. Il Duce — **Benito Mussolini**

15. The Duke — **John Wayne**

16. Scarface — **Al Capone**

17. The Desert Fox — **Erwin Rommel**

18. Ol' Blue Eyes — **Frank Sinatra**

19. Superman — **Clark Kent**

20. Schnozzola — **Jimmy Durante**

FACILITATOR: *Nicknames go back thousands of years. No doubt many people in the group have nicknames. Ask participants for their nicknames, where the nicknames came from, and whether they like the nicknames. Can they think of other famous people who have nicknames by which they are better known? What other items (e.g., places, animals, events) have nicknames?*

Occupations of Famous People

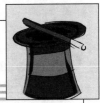

Famous people are known for many reasons—which families they came from, what they invented, the positions they held in politics, or special feats they performed. Perhaps more than anything, though, they are known for their occupations. Match the occupations on the left with the famous people who worked in that occupation on the right.

___ 1. Anthropologist

___ 2. Violin maker

___ 3. Bicyclist

___ 4. Painter

___ 5. Guide and interpreter

___ 6. Architect

___ 7. Mathematician and physicist

___ 8. Opera singer

___ 9. Professional golfer

___ 10. U.S. ambassador

___ 11. Supreme court justice

___ 12. Explorer

___ 13. Astronaut

___ 14. Markswoman

___ 15. Nun

___ 16. Newspaper publisher

___ 17. Magician

___ 18. Spy

___ 19. Journalist and writer

___ 20. Nurse

a. William Randolph Hearst

b. Shirley Temple Black

c. Albert Einstein

d. Clara Barton

e. Annie Oakley

f. Mother Teresa

g. Samuel Clemens (Mark Twain)

h. Ferdinand Magellan

i. Margaret Mead

j. "Babe" Didrikson Zaharias

k. Mata Hari

l. Sandra Day O'Connor

m. Lance Armstrong

n. Sacagawea

o. Frank Lloyd Wright

p. "Grandma" Moses

q. Marian Anderson

r. Harry Houdini

s. Antonio Stradivari

t. Sally Ride

Occupations of Famous People ANSWER SHEET

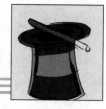

1. Anthropologist   i. **Margaret Mead**

2. Violin maker   s. **Antonio Stradivari**

3. Bicyclist   m. **Lance Armstrong**

4. Painter   p. **"Grandma" Moses**

5. Guide and interpreter   n. **Sacagawea**

6. Architect   o. **Frank Lloyd Wright**

7. Mathematician and physicist   c. **Albert Einstein**

8. Opera singer   q. **Marian Anderson**

9. Professional golfer   j. **"Babe" Didrikson Zaharias**

10. U.S. ambassador   b. **Shirley Temple Black**

11. Supreme court justice   l. **Sandra Day O'Connor**

12. Explorer   h. **Ferdinand Magellan**

13. Astronaut   t. **Sally Ride**

14. Markswoman   e. **Annie Oakley**

15. Nun   f. **Mother Teresa**

16. Newspaper publisher   a. **William Randolph Hearst**

17. Magician   r. **Harry Houdini**

18. Spy   k. **Mata Hari**

19. Journalist and writer   g. **Samuel Clemens (Mark Twain)**

20. Nurse   d. **Clara Barton**

FACILITATOR: *After reviewing the correct answers, discuss the lives of these famous people and what made them famous. Ask participants the following questions: Who are some other famous people with these occupations? Which of these famous people were also rich? What did it take to become rich? Which of these occupations sounds most exciting?*

Occupations Throughout the Ages

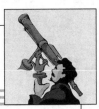

The number of occupation titles has continually expanded over hundreds of years. Today, there are literally thousands of job titles. Below are just a few of those, many of which are named after the sciences. Match the description on the left with the occupation on the right.

___ 1. This person studies past human life and culture.

___ 2. This person studies the origin, behavior, and cultural development of man.

___ 3. This person is in charge of an institution such as a museum.

___ 4. This person studies animals and animal life.

___ 5. This person is a mapmaker.

___ 6. This person studies plants.

___ 7. This person studies life in prehistoric times.

___ 8. This person studies the origin, history, and structure of the earth.

___ 9. This person records in writing.

___ 10. This official maintains order in a courtroom.

___ 11. This person creates and arranges dances.

___ 12. This person studies insects.

___ 13. This person writes the words to songs.

___ 14. This person cares for trees.

___ 15. This person studies the climate.

___ 16. This person studies hearing and hearing defects.

___ 17. This person is a high-ranking administrative official.

___ 18. This person studies earthquakes.

___ 19. This person is the leader of a Jewish congregation.

___ 20. This person deals in men's furnishings.

a. Arborist

b. Transcriptionist

c. Geologist

d. Paleontologist

e. Lyricist

f. Seismologist

g. Entomologist

h. Archaeologist

i. Anthropologist

j. Rabbi

k. Haberdasher

l. Cartographer

m. Climatologist

n. Zoologist

o. Bailiff

p. Botanist

q. Audiologist

r. Curator

s. Choreographer

t. Provost

Occupations Throughout the Ages ANSWER SHEET

1. This person studies past human life and culture.   h.   **Archaeologist**

2. This person studies the origin, behavior, and cultural development of man.   i.   **Anthropologist**

3. This person is in charge of an institution such as a museum.   r.   **Curator**

4. This person studies animals and animal life.   n.   **Zoologist**

5. This person is a mapmaker.   l.   **Cartographer**

6. This person studies plants.   p.   **Botanist**

7. This person studies life in prehistoric times.   d.   **Paleontologist**

8. This person studies the origin, history, and structure of the earth.   c.   **Geologist**

9. This person records in writing.   b.   **Transcriptionist**

10. This official maintains order in a courtroom.   o.   **Bailiff**

11. This person creates and arranges dances.   s.   **Choreographer**

12. This person studies insects.   g.   **Entomologist**

13. This person writes the words to songs.   e.   **Lyricist**

14. This person cares for trees.   a.   **Arborist**

15. This person studies the climate.   m.   **Climatologist**

16. This person studies hearing and hearing defects.   q.   **Audiologist**

17. This person is a high-ranking administrative official.   t.   **Provost**

18. This person studies earthquakes.   f.   **Seismologist**

19. This person is the leader of a Jewish congregation.   j.   **Rabbi**

20. This person deals in men's furnishings.   k.   **Haberdasher**

FACILITATOR: *Once this worksheet is completed, possible topics for discussion with participants include the following: What did you do for a living? What was your favorite job? What were the wages then versus now? How have occupations changed over the years? Are wages fair? How do occupations compare against each other (a professional baseball star versus a secretary)? What, if given a choice, would you do for a living now?*

Strengthen Your Mind by Einberger & Sellick. © 2007 by Health Professions Press, Inc.

Personalities in Advertising

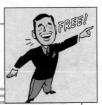

The famous Oscar Mayer Wienermobile began advertising in 1936, complete with Wiener Whistles. Other "personalities" began even earlier, all with the attempt to lure customers to use their products. Use the following clues to name the advertising personalities described.

1. What jolly, rotund figure has advertised tires since 1898?

2. What green, larger-than-life figure from the valley has advertised a variety of vegetables since 1928?

3. Which cat advertises 9Lives Cat Food?

4. Which man, wearing a white chef's hat, has his face on a red-and-white label advertising cheap pasta with tomato sauce?

5. What plump white figure began advertising "poppin' fresh" baking products in the 1960s?

6. Who has adorned pancake mix and syrup since 1893, though her appearance has changed radically to be more socially appropriate?

7. Kellogg's Frosted Flakes are promoted by which animal, who has a trademark growl of "They're grrrreat!"?

8. Which genie-looking man advertises products for household cleaning?

9. Which animal keeps going and going and going while advertising batteries?

10. Which happy female cow began advertising Borden dairy products in 1939?

11. In 1955, this cowboy, the epitome of masculinity, began advertising cigarettes?

12. Which clown advertises for the Golden Arches?

13. Which large animal serves as a symbol for the U.S. Forest Service, warning, "Only you can prevent forest fires!"?

14. Which figure, with a hat and cane, was created for Planters in 1916?

15. Which imaginary lady has advertised bakery goods, especially cake mixes, and "authored" cookbooks for General Mills since 1921?

16. Which majestic horses have been a symbol for Anheuser-Busch for more than 75 years?

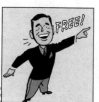

Personalities in Advertising ANSWER SHEET

1. What jolly, rotund figure has advertised tires since 1898?
   The Michelin Man

2. What green, larger-than-life figure from the valley has advertised a variety of vegetables since 1928?
   The Green Giant

3. Which cat advertises 9Lives Cat Food?
   Morris

4. Which man, wearing a white chef's hat, has his face on a red-and-white label advertising cheap pasta with tomato sauce?
   Chef Boyardee

5. What plump white figure began advertising "poppin' fresh" baking products in the 1960s?
   Pillsbury Doughboy

6. Who has adorned pancake mix and syrup since 1893, though her appearance has changed radically to be more socially appropriate?
   Aunt Jemima

7. Kellogg's Frosted Flakes are promoted by which animal, who has a trademark growl of "They're grrrreat!"?
   Tony the Tiger

8. Which genie-looking man advertises products for household cleaning?
   Mr. Clean

9. Which animal keeps going and going and going while advertising batteries?
   Energizer Bunny

10. Which happy female cow began advertising Borden dairy products in 1939?
    Elsie

11. In 1955, this cowboy, the epitome of masculinity, began advertising cigarettes?
    The Marlboro Man

12. Which clown advertises for the Golden Arches?
    Ronald McDonald

13. Which large animal serves as a symbol for the U.S. Forest Service, warning, "Only you can prevent forest fires!"?
    Smokey the Bear

14. Which figure, with a hat and cane, was created for Planters in 1916?
    Mr. Peanut

15. Which imaginary lady has advertised bakery goods, especially cake mixes, and "authored" cookbooks for General Mills since 1921?
    Betty Crocker

16. Which majestic horses have been a symbol for Anheuser-Busch for more than 75 years?
    The Clydesdales

FACILITATOR: *These larger-than-life personalities are sure to bring up many memories. Ask participants who has used each product. What other personalities are used to promote products? If participants were to create a personality for advertising, what would it be?*

Strengthen Your Mind by Einberger & Sellick. © 2007 by Health Professions Press, Inc.

Pets of Fame

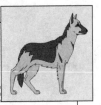

Although most of us have had pets that we hold dear, the pets listed on this sheet were not only companions but stars as well. Some were movie stars, some were television stars, and some even lived in the White House. Read the clues on the left and match them with the correct answer on the right.

___ 1. This famous talking horse starred in his own 1960s television show with his owner, Wilbur.

___ 2. This German shepherd made the breed famous and was the nation's first canine movie star after a role in the silent movie *The Man from Hell's River*.

___ 3. This comic strip, written by Jim Davis, starred a fat orange cat with lots of attitude and a big appetite.

___ 4. This 1995 movie about a pig raised by sheep-dogs that learned to herd sheep himself made its loveable main character famous.

___ 5. Socks was the name of this president's black and white cat that lived in the White House with his brother, Buddy, a chocolate lab.

___ 6. Originally a book character, this dog is America's most favorite collie and has spent more than 50 years on television.

___ 7. This beagle and his owner, Charlie Brown, starred in the comic strip by Charles Schultz.

___ 8. Since 1974, this loveable dog has starred in numerous television shows and movies after being adopted from an animal shelter.

___ 9. This 1950s television show featured "King of the Cowboys" Roy Rogers and this horse, the "Smartest Horse in the Movies."

___ 10. In this late 1960s television series, a young boy befriends a bear cub and convinces his father to purchase the cub for a pet.

___ 11. This president had a mongrel dog named Yuki that was a star in the White House. The two loved to perform by "singing" together for visitors.

___ 12. Perhaps one of the most famous racehorses of all time, this champion won the Triple Crown in 1973, the first horse to do so in 25 years.

___ 13. This 1993 movie foreshadowed the real-life story of a whale named Keiko that was returned to the wild.

___ 14. This loveable bear became famous for teaching young children about the importance of preventing forest fires.

a. *Free Willy*

b. Trigger

c. President Johnson

d. *Gentle Ben*

e. *Babe*

f. Rin Tin Tin

g. Mr. Ed

h. Garfield

i. President Clinton

j. Snoopy

k. Smokey the Bear

l. Benji

m. Lassie

n. Secretariat

Pets of Fame ANSWER SHEET

1. This famous talking horse starred in his own 1960s television show with his owner, Wilbur.

   g.   **Mr. Ed**

2. This German shepherd made the breed famous and was the nation's first canine movie star after a role in the silent movie *The Man from Hell's River.*

   f.   **Rin Tin Tin**

3. This comic strip, written by Jim Davis, starred a fat orange cat with lots of attitude and a big appetite.

   h.   **Garfield**

4. This 1995 movie about a pig raised by sheepdogs that learned to herd sheep himself made its loveable main character famous.

   e.   ***Babe***

5. Socks was the name of this president's black and white cat that lived in the White House with his brother, Buddy, a chocolate lab.

   i.   **President Clinton**

6. Originally a book character, this dog is America's most favorite collie and has spent more than 50 years on television.

   m.   **Lassie**

7. This beagle and his owner, Charlie Brown, starred in the comic strip by Charles Schultz.

   j.   **Snoopy**

8. Since 1974, this loveable dog has starred in numerous television shows and movies after being adopted from an animal shelter.

   l.   **Benji**

9. This 1950s television show featured "King of the Cowboys" Roy Rogers and this horse, the "Smartest Horse in the Movies."

   b.   **Trigger**

10. In this late 1960s television series, a young boy befriends a bear cub and convinces his father to purchase the cub for a pet.

   d.   ***Gentle Ben***

11. This president had a mongrel dog named Yuki that was a star in the White House. The two loved to perform by "singing" together for visitors.

   c.   **President Johnson**

12. Perhaps one of the most famous racehorses of all time, this champion won the Triple Crown in 1973, the first horse to do so in 25 years.

   n.   **Secretariat**

13. This 1993 movie foreshadowed the real-life story of a whale named Keiko that was returned to the wild.

   a.   ***Free Willy***

14. This loveable bear became famous for teaching young children about the importance of preventing forest fires.

   k.   **Smokey the Bear**

FACILITATOR: *There are many more famous animals that have appeared in film and television. Encourage participants to name as many as they can. Ask the following questions: Did you watch the shows or movies listed on this worksheet? Can you name any additional presidential pets? What qualities make an animal appropriate for television? For fun, ask participants what trick they would teach an animal if the animal were able to learn anything.*

Queens, Kings, and Other Royalty

Royalty has been a subject of fascination for hundreds of years. Queens and kings still reign in approximately 30 monarchies throughout the world. Some have real power; others are simply figureheads. Identify the following royal things.

1. Which former actress married the Prince of Monaco?

2. Which queen of England reigned for nearly 64 years, longer than any other?

3. William Shakespeare flourished during the reign of which monarch, also known as the Virgin Queen?

4. Wallis Simpson's love affair with which king forced him to abdicate the throne in 1936?

5. Which English king married six times and had two of his wives executed for infidelity?

6. Legendary stories of which king include the characters of Lancelot and Guinevere?

7. Yul Brynner portrayed which king in *The King and I*?

8. Name Queen Elizabeth II's children.

9. Which building is the Queen's official London residence?

10. HRH, Duchess of Cornwall is which lady's title? (*Hint:* She is Prince Charles's second wife.)

11. Which young king, who died around 1343 B.C., was buried in a now-famous tomb, which was found in nearly perfect condition?

12. Which luxury liner, named after a famous queen, now serves as a hotel in Long Beach, California?

13. Queen Elizabeth is referred to as "HM," and her husband, Prince Philip, as "HRH." What do these stand for?

14. Since 1303, which collection of ceremonial regalia, including coronation crowns, has been housed in the Tower of London?

15. Which castle, the largest occupied castle in the world, serves as a retreat for the Queen of England and is just a few miles from London?

1. Which former actress married the Prince of Monaco?
   Princess Grace

2. Which queen of England reigned for nearly 64 years, longer than any other?
   Queen Victoria

3. William Shakespeare flourished during the reign of which monarch, also known as the Virgin Queen?
   Queen Elizabeth I

4. Wallis Simpson's love affair with which king forced him to abdicate the throne in 1936?
   King Edward VIII

5. Which English king married six times and had two of his wives executed for infidelity?
   Henry VIII

6. Legendary stories of which king include the characters Lancelot and Guinevere?
   King Arthur

7. Yul Brynner portrayed which king in *The King and I*?
   King of Siam

8. Name Queen Elizabeth II's children.
   Prince Charles, Princess Anne, Prince Andrew, Prince Edward

9. Which building is the Queen's official London residence?
   Buckingham Palace

10. HRH, Duchess of Cornwall is which lady's title? (*Hint:* She is Prince Charles's second wife.)
    Camilla Parker Bowles

11. Which young king, who died around 1343 B.C., was buried in a now-famous tomb, which was found in nearly perfect condition?
    King Tut

12. Which luxury liner, named after a famous queen, now serves as a hotel in Long Beach, California?
    RMS Queen Mary

13. Queen Elizabeth is referred to as "HM," and her husband, Prince Philip, as "HRH." What do these stand for?
    Her Majesty, His Royal Highness

14. Since 1303, which collection of ceremonial regalia, including coronation crowns, has been housed in the Tower of London?
    Crown Jewels

15. Which castle, the largest occupied castle in the world, serves as a retreat for the Queen of England and is just a few miles from London?
    Windsor Castle

FACILITATOR: *Going through each question will afford great opportunities for discussion. Which participants would like to be kings or queens? How would life be different? Does the British system of having both a queen and a prime minister make sense? Would the billions of dollars spent on British royalty be better spent elsewhere? Who are other famous kings and queens? What would it be like to live in a castle and be surrounded by your own guards? What would it be like to be married into royalty?*

Quotes that Made History

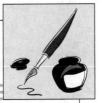

Quotes from famous people have been known to have a profound impact on the history of the world. Other quotes cause us to ponder the past, the present, and the future. Still others offer us inspiration and humor. Match the quote on the left with the author on the right.

___ 1. I have a dream . . .

___ 2. I only regret that I have but one life to lose for my country.

___ 3. Ask not what your country can do for you— ask what you can do for your country.

___ 4. I'm not a crook!

___ 5. Between two evils, I always pick the one I never tried before.

___ 6. Genius is one percent inspiration, ninety-nine percent perspiration.

___ 7. The buck stops here.

___ 8. Frankly, my dear, I don't give a damn.

___ 9. Speak softly and carry a big stick.

___ 10. Any customer can have a car painted any color that he wants so long as it is black.

___ 11. The only thing we have to fear is fear itself.

___ 12. Housework can't kill you but why take a chance?

___ 13. Never doubt that a small group of thoughtful, committed citizens can change the world, indeed it is the only thing that ever has.

___ 14. No one can make you feel inferior without your consent.

___ 15. I shall return.

___ 16. I never met a man I didn't like.

___ 17. History will be kind to me, for I intend to write it.

___ 18. I have everything I had 20 years ago except now it's all lower.

___ 19. That's one small step for man, one giant leap for mankind.

a. Eleanor Roosevelt

b. Clark Gable (as Rhett Butler)

c. Martin Luther King, Jr.

d. Mae West (as The Frisco Doll)

e. Neil Armstrong

f. Franklin Delano Roosevelt

g. Richard Nixon

h. Theodore Roosevelt

i. Nathan Hale

j. Will Rogers

k. Gypsy Rose Lee

l. Henry Ford

m. Douglas MacArthur

n. Harry Truman

o. John F. Kennedy

p. Thomas Edison

q. Phyllis Diller

r. Margaret Mead

s. Sir Winston Churchill

Quotes that Made History ANSWER SHEET

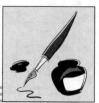

1. I have a dream . . .   **c.**   **Martin Luther King, Jr.**

2. I only regret that I have but one life to lose for my country.   **i.**   **Nathan Hale**

3. Ask not what your country can do for you—ask what you can do for your country.   **o.**   **John F. Kennedy**

4. I'm not a crook!   **g.**   **Richard Nixon**

5. Between two evils, I always pick the one I never tried before.   **d.**   **Mae West (as The Frisco Doll)**

6. Genius is one percent inspiration, ninety-nine percent perspiration.   **p.**   **Thomas Edison**

7. The buck stops here.   **n.**   **Harry Truman**

8. Frankly, my dear, I don't give a damn.   **b.**   **Clark Gable (as Rhett Butler)**

9. Speak softly and carry a big stick.   **h.**   **Theodore Roosevelt**

10. Any customer can have a car painted any color that he wants so long as it is black.   **l.**   **Henry Ford**

11. The only thing we have to fear is fear itself.   **f.**   **Franklin Delano Roosevelt**

12. Housework can't kill you but why take a chance?   **q.**   **Phyllis Diller**

13. Never doubt that a small group of thoughtful, committed citizens can change the world, indeed it is the only thing that ever has.   **r.**   **Margaret Mead**

14. No one can make you feel inferior without your consent.   **a.**   **Eleanor Roosevelt**

15. I shall return.   **m.**   **Douglas MacArthur**

16. I never met a man I didn't like.   **j.**   **Will Rogers**

17. History will be kind to me, for I intend to write it.   **s.**   **Sir Winston Churchill**

18. I have everything I had 20 years ago except now it's all lower.   **k.**   **Gypsy Rose Lee**

19. That's one small step for man, one giant leap for mankind.   **e.**   **Neil Armstrong**

FACILITATOR: As participants complete this worksheet, ask them to reflect on each quote and the person who said it. Are the quotes meaningful in participants' lives? Do participants respect the people who said the quotes? Do the quotes really reflect the lives that the people who spoke them lived? Ask participants for other meaningful quotes. Explore how it is that some quotes make history and others are never repeated. Is it because of the author, the meaning, or the situation?

Radio's Golden Years

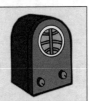

Radio has long been one of the most popular entertainment choices for American families. From its humble beginnings to the technological advances of today, radio has been a source of entertainment, news, and connection with the world. Answer the following questions about radio's Golden Years.

1. Which comedy program was the first serial created for radio and starred two friends who moved to Chicago and started their own taxi company?

2. Which president is famous for his evening "Fireside Chats" on the radio from 1933 to 1945?

3. Which program caused widespread panic in 1938 when listeners thought a dramatization of H.G. Wells's fantasy book was a real newscast?

4. Which tune by Bing Crosby is the number one recorded song on radio and has sold more than 35 million copies since it was recorded in 1942?

5. The "simple, wholesome times" that signified the height of radio popularity were from about 1929 to 1957 and are often called what? (*Hint:* The _____ of Radio.)

6. Which radio program starring a cowboy and his horse, Silver, began in 1933 and spawned numerous comic books, movies, and a television series?

7. Which late 1970s television show starring Andy Travis was about employees at a Cincinnati radio station and their gimmicks to make the station successful?

8. Which radio comedy program ran from the 1930s until the 1950s, when it became a hit television show? (*Hint:* It starred one of the most famous comedy duos of all time, ditzy Gracie and her husband, George.)

9. On Christmas Eve 1906 in Brandt Rock, Massachusetts, the first what was played over the radio?

10. From 1941 to 1952, which suspense radio program thrilled listeners with its trademark "creaking" door that began and ended each show?

11. Who used a variety of household items to make sounds during radio programs?

12. Finish the catchphrase of this 1930s detective radio program: "Who knows what evil lurks in the hearts of men? The _____ knows!"

13. Which famous radio personality is known as the King of the Countdowns for the *American Top 40* that began in 1970?

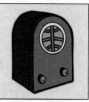

Radio's Golden Years ANSWER SHEET

1. Which comedy program was the first serial created for radio and starred two friends who moved to Chicago and started their own taxi company?
   Amos 'n' Andy

2. Which president is famous for his evening "Fireside Chats" on the radio from 1933 to 1945?
   Franklin D. Roosevelt

3. Which program caused widespread panic in 1938 when listeners thought a dramatization of H.G. Wells's fantasy book was a real newscast?
   The War of the Worlds

4. Which tune by Bing Crosby is the number one recorded song on radio and has sold more than 35 million copies since it was recorded in 1942?
   White Christmas

5. The "simple, wholesome times" that signified the height of radio popularity were from about 1929 to 1957 and are often called what? (*Hint:* The _____ of Radio.)
   Golden Years or Golden Age

6. Which radio program starring a cowboy and his horse, Silver, began in 1933 and spawned numerous comic books, movies, and a television series?
   The Lone Ranger

7. Which late 1970s television show starring Andy Travis was about employees at a Cincinnati radio station and their gimmicks to make the station successful?
   WKRP in Cincinnati

8. Which radio comedy program ran from the 1930s until the 1950s, when it became a hit television show? (*Hint:* It starred one of the most famous comedy duos of all time, ditzy Gracie and her husband, George.)
   Burns and Allen

9. On Christmas Eve 1906 in Brandt Rock, Massachusetts, the first what was played over the radio?
   Song

10. From 1941 to 1952, which suspense radio program thrilled listeners with its trademark "creaking" door that began and ended each show?
    Inner Sanctum Mysteries

11. Who used a variety of household items to make sounds during radio programs?
    Sound man

12. Finish the catchphrase of this 1930s detective radio program: "Who knows what evil lurks in the hearts of men? The _____ knows!"
    Shadow

13. Which famous radio personality is known as the King of the Countdowns for hosting the *American Top 40* that began in 1970?
    Casey Kasem

FACILITATOR: *Radio is a great discussion topic. Ask participants to name additional radio programs from the Golden Age (e.g., Lum and Abner, Fibber McGee and Molly, The Great Gildersleeve, The $64,000 Question). Try to find a recording of an episode for discussion. How do the radio programs of today differ? What program marked the end of radio's Golden Age? (Answer: CBS broadcasts of Suspense and Yours Truly, Johnny Dollar on September 30, 1962).*

Red, White, and Blue

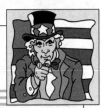

Red, white, and blue have a longstanding significance to the United States. Not only are these the colors of our flag, but they are also used for many of our symbols and celebrations, such as the Fourth of July. The following clues all relate to these colors or to other symbols, events, and facts in U.S. history. Identify the items described by the clues.

1.   Which U.S. symbol, first made in 1751 and remade several times since, now sits near Independence Hall in Philadelphia?

2.   What is the oldest U.S. military academy?

3.   Name at least two nicknames for the U.S. flag.

4.   What fictitious man has a beard and wears a red, white, and blue suit and hat?

5.   Whose signature became well known for being the largest on the *Declaration of Independence?*

6.   Many students start off their school day by reciting which speech to the flag?

7.   What significant voting event happened on August 18, 1920?

8.   Which bugle call, written in 1862, is often sung at military funerals?

9.   What does the term *G.I.* stand for?

10. Women were recruited to work in factories during World War II, often using the image of which strong woman?

11. What is the name of the presidential airplane?

12. Who entertained U.S. troops for 50 years, many times at Christmas?

13. Which song is sung before most major league baseball games?

14. Name the three branches of government.

15. Name the five branches of the Armed Forces.

16. The structural framework of what monument to freedom was designed by Alexandre Gustave Eiffel, the designer of the Eiffel Tower in Paris?

17. Whose faces appear on Mount Rushmore in South Dakota?

Red, White, and Blue ANSWER SHEET

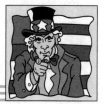

1. Which U.S. symbol, first made in 1751 and remade several times since, now sits near Independence Hall in Philadelphia?
   Liberty Bell

2. What is the oldest U.S. military academy?
   West Point (1802)

3. Name at least two nicknames for the U.S. flag.
   Old Glory; the Red, White, and Blue; the Star-Spangled Banner; Stars and Stripes

4. What fictitious man has a beard and wears a red, white, and blue suit and hat?
   Uncle Sam

5. Whose signature became well known for being the largest on the *Declaration of Independence?*
   John Hancock

6. Many students start off their school day by reciting which speech to the flag?
   Pledge of Allegiance

7. What significant voting event happened on August 18, 1920?
   Ratification of the 19th Amendment, giving women the right to vote

8. Which bugle call, written in 1862, is often played at military funerals?
   Taps

9. What does the term *G.I.* stand for?
   Government issue or general issue

10. Women were recruited to work in factories during World War II, often using the image of which strong woman?
    Rosie the Riveter

11. What is the name of the presidential airplane?
    Air Force One

12. Who entertained U.S. troops for 50 years, many times at Christmas?
    Bob Hope

13. Which song is sung before most major league baseball games?
    The Star Spangled Banner

14. Name the three branches of government.
    Executive, Judicial, Legislative

15. Name the five branches of the Armed Forces.
    Air Force, Army, Coast Guard, Marine Corps, Navy

16. The structural framework of what monument to freedom was designed by Alexandre Gustave Eiffel, the designer of the Eiffel Tower in Paris?
    Statue of Liberty

17. Whose faces appear on Mt. Rushmore in South Dakota?
    Abraham Lincoln, George Washington, Theodore Roosevelt, Thomas Jefferson

FACILITATOR: *These questions are sure to bring up many interesting conversations! Ask participants the following questions: What other symbols represent the United States? Do you feel patriotic when you see these symbols? What about when you see the flag flying or hear the national anthem being sung? Should the Pledge of Allegiance be mandatory? What are your feelings about women's right to vote? What do you think about Bob Hope's 50 years of service to the military? Can you put yourself in his shoes? Whose picture is on the $1 bill? What about the $5 bill, $10 bill, $20 bill, and so forth? Whose picture is on the penny? What about the nickel, dime, and so forth?*

Strengthen Your Mind by Einberger & Sellick. © 2007 by Health Professions Press, Inc.

Spectrum of Color

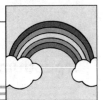

Color can have a very beneficial effect on our memories. When trying to remember something, most of us visualize in color rather than black and white. We constantly use color cues to help us remember someone's name, a place we have visited, and more. Answer the following questions dealing with color to the best of your ability.

1. What acronym represents the colors of the rainbow?

2. What are the original eight colors of Crayola crayons? (Today, Crayola crayons come in 120 core colors.)

3. What are the primary colors?

4. What are the secondary colors?

5. Name three different shades of red.

6. Which three seas are named after colors?

7. What was the most popular car color from 2000 to 2005?

8. Which color is on the top of a stoplight?

9. Which color is the top stripe of the U.S. flag? (*Bonus:* What do each of the colors stand for?)

10. What are the colors of the French flag?

11. What are the colors of the Canadian flag?

12. What are the colors of the Japanese flag?

13. What are the colors of the flag of the United Kingdom?

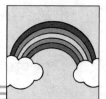

1. What acronym represents the colors of the rainbow?
    ROYGBIV

2. What are the original eight colors of Crayola crayons? (Today, Crayola crayons come in 120 core colors.)
    Black, blue, brown, green, orange, red, violet, yellow

3. What are the primary colors?
    Blue, red, yellow

4. What are the secondary colors?
    Green, orange, purple (violet)

5. Name three different shades of red.
    Apple, beet, brick, burgundy, cardinal, cinnabar, crimson, fire engine, fuchsia, maroon, pink, plum, rouge, ruby, scarlet, vermillion

6. Which three seas are named after colors?
    Black Sea, Red Sea, Yellow Sea

7. What was the most popular car color from 2000 to 2005?
    Silver

8. Which color is on the top of a stoplight?
    Red

9. Which color is the top stripe of the U.S. flag? (*Bonus:* What do the colors stand for?)
    Red (Blue: vigilance, perseverance, and justice; red: valor and bravery; white: purity and innocence)

10. What are the colors of the French flag?
    Blue, red, white

11. What are the colors of the Canadian flag?
    Red, white

12. What are the colors of the Japanese flag?
    Red, white

13. What are the colors of the flag of the United Kingdom?
    Blue, red, white

FACILITATOR: *These questions will probably bring up many memories, from the first time participants colored with crayons to the color of their first cars. Ask participants to expand on their answers to include their own thoughts. Name shades of different colors. What are participants' favorite colors? The possibilities of discussion on the topic of color are endless.*

Strengthen Your Mind by Einberger & Sellick. © 2007 by Health Professions Press, Inc.

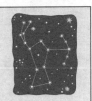

Stars of the Universe

Stars are usually a sign of something good, of something "heavenly." The following facts all describe things that contain the word *star*. Identify each one.

1. What is another name for the American flag?

2. What is the brightest star in Ursa Minor, or the Little Dipper?

3. What emblem symbolizes Judaism?

4. Finish the song lyric: "_____ _____, _____ _____, first star I see tonight."

5. What is the name of the famous nursery rhyme that contains the lyrics "like a diamond in the sky"?

6. What is the right side of a ship called?

7. Name one of the nation's most well-known coffee chains.

8. A top-notch hotel is called what?

9. What is a streak of light in the sky at night caused by a meteor called?

10. The best performer, such as in sports, is called what?

11. What is the first line from the refrain of *We Three Kings of Orient Are?*

12. Name a well-known brand of tuna.

13. A sea star is another name for what ocean dweller?

14. Francis Scott Key wrote what? (*Hint:* It is our national anthem.)

15. Bumping one's head and having blurred vision is called what?

16. A dreamlike and romantic quality is called what?

17. To observe the stars or to daydream is called what?

18. What series of movies by Steven Spielberg includes *The Empire Strikes Back* and *Return of the Jedi?*

Stars of the Universe ANSWER SHEET

1. What is another name for the American flag?
    Stars and Stripes, Star-Spangled Banner

2. What is the brightest star in Ursa Minor, or the Little Dipper?
    North star (Polaris)

3. What emblem symbolizes Judaism?
    Star of David

4. Finish this song lyric: "_____ _____, _____ _____, first star I see tonight."
    Star light, star bright

5. What is the name of the famous nursery rhyme that contains the lyrics "like a diamond in the sky"?
    "Twinkle, Twinkle Little Star"

6. What is the right side of a ship called?
    Starboard

7. Name one of the nation's most well-known coffee chains.
    Starbucks

8. A top-notch hotel is called what?
    Five-star hotel

9. What is a streak of light in the sky at night caused by a meteor called?
    Shooting star

10. The best performer, such as in sports, is called what?
    All-star

11. What is the first line from the refrain of *We Three Kings of Orient Are*?
    "O star of wonder, star of night"

12. Name a well-known brand of tuna.
    Starkist tuna

13. A sea star is another name for what ocean dweller?
    Starfish

14. Francis Scott Key wrote what? (*Hint:* It is our national anthem.)
    The Star-Spangled Banner

15. Bumping one's head and having blurred vision is called what?
    Seeing stars

16. A dreamlike and romantic quality is called what?
    Stardust

17. To observe the stars or to daydream is called what?
    Stargaze

18. What series of movies by Steven Spielberg includes *The Empire Strikes Back* and *Return of the Jedi*?
    Star Wars

FACILITATOR: *When we think of stars, many definitions come to mind—the stars in the sky, a star athlete or movie star, a shape of a piece of jewelry. Discuss the above words and phrases with participants. Ask the following questions: What other brands of tuna are there? What other songs have "star" in the lyrics? Who are the greatest superstars? Have you stayed in a five-star hotel? What other well-known phrases contain the word "star"? Do you stargaze?*

Strengthen Your Mind by Einberger & Sellick. © 2007 by Health Professions Press, Inc.

Television Quotes—Famous Lines of Famous Stars

Most of us have been watching television for more than 50 years. Some shows remain etched in our minds; some are easily forgotten. This is true of the stars of these shows, too. Certainly some are memorable. Each of the following lines was said on a well-known television show by a famous star. Name the star, either by the television character's name or the actor's real name.

1. Good night, Mrs. Calabash, wherever you are.

2. Heeeeeeere's Johnny!

3. Well, golly!

4. Lucy, you got some 'splainin' to do.

5. And a one, and a two . . .

6. Good night, and may God bless.

7. We're going to have a really good "shew."

8. One of these days, Alice . . .

9. Hi-yo Silver, away!

10. Just the facts, ma'am.

11. Yabba dabba doo

12. Say goodnight, Gracie.

13. I don't get no respect.

14. Good night, David . . . Good night, Chet.

15. Wonderful, wonderful. (Wunnerful, wunnerful.)

16. Come on down.

17. This is your life.

18. Happy trails to you, until we meet again . . .

Television Quotes—
Famous Lines of Famous Stars ANSWER SHEET

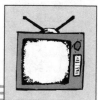

1. Good night, Mrs. Calabash, wherever you are.
   Jimmy Durante

2. Heeeeeeere's Johnny!
   Ed McMahon (on *The Tonight Show starring Johnny Carson*)

3. Well, golly!
   Jim Nabors as Gomer Pyle

4. Lucy, you got some 'splainin' to do.
   Desi Arnaz as Ricky Ricardo

5. And a one, and a two . . .
   Lawrence Welk

6. Good night, and may God bless.
   Red Skelton

7. We're going to have a really good "shew."
   Ed Sullivan

8. One of these days, Alice . . .
   Jackie Gleason as Ralph Kramden

9. Hi-yo Silver, away!
   Clayton Moore as The Lone Ranger

10. Just the facts, ma'am.
    Jack Webb as Sgt. Joe Friday

11. Yabba dabba doo
    Fred Flintstone

12. Say goodnight, Gracie.
    George Burns

13. I don't get no respect.
    Rodney Dangerfield

14. Good night, David . . . Good night, Chet
    David Brinkley and Chet Huntley

15. Wonderful, wonderful. (Wunnerful, wunnerful.)
    Lawrence Welk

16. Come on down.
    Bob Barker on *The Price is Right*

17. This is your life.
    Ralph Edwards

18. Happy trails to you, until we meet again . . .
    Dale Evans and Roy Rogers

FACILITATOR: *This activity is great for a lot of conversation. Participants can discuss each star, the television show, the other stars on the show, other shows and movies that the stars appeared in, and a comparison of television today with television of the 1950s, 1960s, and so forth. Ask participants for their favorite television shows and favorite stars. What shows do they watch today? How many hours of television do they watch? Is it too much? Does it keep them from getting enough exercise?*

Strengthen Your Mind by Einberger & Sellick. © 2007 by Health Professions Press, Inc.

Time and Time Again

We depend on time for much of what we do. What time is dinner? What time is our doctor's appointment? What time is the movie? What time are our guests coming for dinner? And, of course, most of us would love more than 24 hours in our days! Match the description on the left with the answer containing the word *time* on the right.

___ 1. This time system "saves" daylight.

___ 2. To be slow or dawdle is to do this.

___ 3. This is another word for universal time.

___ 4. This time system uses a 24-hour clock, rather than A.M. and P.M.

___ 5. This is one of the most well-known weekly news magazines.

___ 6. This means to do something aimless in order to pass time.

___ 7. This is a large East Coast daily newspaper.

___ 8. This is the amount of time between when something is ordered and when it is completed.

___ 9. This is the rate of pay that people earn when they work overtime.

___ 10. This famous landmark in New York City is home to theaters, restaurants, and many, many lights.

___ 11. A short, requested break in a sports game is called this.

___ 12. This receptacle contains articles from a particular time period that may be opened in the future.

___ 13. This machine records when an employee checks in and out of work.

___ 14. Something that is eternal or everlasting is called this.

___ 15. There are 24 of these longitudinal divisions around the world.

___ 16. Another name for a watch or clock is this.

___ 17. When a person works 40 hours per week, he or she is said to work this.

a.   Lead-time

b.   Time and a half

c.   Time out

d.   Timepiece

e.   Time capsule

f.   Timeless

g.   Time zones

h.   Times Square

i.   Daylight Savings Time

j.   Full time

k.   Kill time

l.   Military time

m.   *The New York Times*

n.   *Time Magazine*

o.   Greenwich Mean Time

p.   Take one's time

q.   Time clock

Time and Time Again ANSWER SHEET

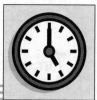

1. This time system "saves" daylight.

    i.   **Daylight Savings Time**

2. To be slow or dawdle is to do this.

    p.   **Take one's time**

3. This is another word for universal time.

    o.   **Greenwich Mean Time**

4. This time system uses a 24-hour clock, rather than A.M. and P.M.

    l.   **Military Time**

5. This is one of the most well-known weekly news magazines.

    n.   *Time Magazine*

6. This means to do something aimless in order to pass time.

    k.   **Kill time**

7. This is a large East Coast daily newspaper.

    m.   *The New York Times*

8. This is the amount of time between when something is ordered and when it is completed.

    a.   **Lead-time**

9. This is the rate of pay that people earn when they work overtime.

    b.   **Time and a half**

10. This famous landmark in New York City is home to theaters, restaurants, and many, many lights.

    h.   **Times Square**

11. A short, requested break in a sports game is called this.

    c.   **Time out**

12. This receptacle contains articles from a particular time period that may be opened in the future.

    e.   **Time capsule**

13. This machine records when an employee checks in and out of work.

    q.   **Time clock**

14. Something that is eternal or everlasting is called this.

    f.   **Timeless**

15. There are 24 of these longitudinal divisions around the world.

    g.   **Time zones**

16. Another name for a watch or clock is this.

    d.   **Timepiece**

17. When a person works 40 hours per week, he or she is said to work this.

    j.   **Full time**

FACILITATOR: *Nearly everyone has something to say about time—there's not enough of it, it passes too quickly, it "stands still." Discuss each phrase as you review the answers. Ask participants the following questions: Would it be easier to keep track of time using military time? Should a standard workweek be 40 hours? Does Time Magazine do a good job of reporting the news? Other areas to explore may be whether or not participants wear watches or have enough time to do all they want to do.*

     Strengthen Your Mind by Einberger & Sellick. © 2007 by Health Professions Press, Inc.

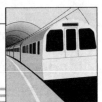

Underground Life

Many types of life exist below us, from animals, to people, to plants. Take a journey below the earth's surface and learn about life underground while answering these questions.

1. In which city will your find the "tube," the oldest underground transportation network in the world?

2. Which trees with shallow, aggressive roots can reach up to 375 feet and are the largest in the world?

3. In the 1800s, Harriet Tubman led thousands of slaves to freedom through which risky route?

4. Which cave located in Southern New Mexico is famous for its gigantic underground chamber?

5. After a thorough cleaning, these vegetables taste great! Name at least five vegetables that grow underground.

6. Which animal, also called a woodchuck, lives underground and makes an appearance each February to tell us if there will be 6 more weeks of winter?

7. What icicle-shaped formations grow when water slowly drips from the ceiling in a cave?

8. We live on top of the Earth's crust. Name the two other layers that begin underneath the crust.

9. Which tiny creatures live in colonies underground and are led by a queen, who spends her life laying eggs?

10. Which underground tunnel reaches across the English Channel from England to France?

11. Many animals go underground during winter to do what in order to conserve energy for the spring?

12. Name five animals that live underground.

13. If you dig far enough into the ground, you will hit the point at which the soil is completely saturated with water, which is called what?

14. At more than 33 miles long, which undersea tunnel is the longest in the world and connects two of Japan's largest islands?

Underground Life ANSWER SHEET

1. In which city will you find the "tube," the oldest underground transportation network in the world?
   London

2. Which trees with shallow, aggressive roots can reach up to 375 feet and are the largest in the world?
   Redwood trees

3. In the 1800s, Harriet Tubman led thousands of slaves to freedom through which risky route?
   Underground Railroad

4. Which cave located in Southern New Mexico is famous for its gigantic underground chamber?
   Carlsbad Caverns

5. After a thorough cleaning, these vegetables taste great! Name at least five vegetables that grow underground.
   Beet, carrot, garlic, onion, potato, radish, turnip, yam

6. Which animal, also called a woodchuck, lives underground and makes an appearance each February to tell us if there will be 6 more weeks of winter?
   Groundhog

7. What icicle-shaped formations grow when water slowly drips from the ceiling in a cave?
   Stalactites

8. We live on top of the Earth's crust. Name the two other layers that begin underneath the crust.
   Core, mantle

9. Which tiny creatures live in colonies underground and are led by a queen, who spends her life laying eggs?
   Ants

10. Which underground tunnel reaches across the English Channel from England to France?
    Chunnel (Channel Tunnel)

11. Many animals go underground during winter to do what in order to conserve energy for the spring?
    Hibernate

12. Name five animals that live underground.
    Aardvark, ants, armadillo, badger, chipmunk, cicada, fox, groundhog, mole, prairie dog, rabbit, shrew, worm

13. If you dig far enough into the ground, you will hit the point at which the soil is completely saturated with water, which is called what?
    Water table

14. At more than 33 miles long, which undersea tunnel is the longest in the world and connects two of Japan's largest islands?
    Seikan Tunnel

FACILITATOR: *Going underground can be fascinating. Ask participants if they have ever been in a cave, under the ocean, or in a tunnel. What does being underground feel like? For further activity, list famous caves throughout the world. Talk about underwater caves. How do they differ from others?*

 Strengthen Your Mind by Einberger & Sellick. © 2007 by Health Professions Press, Inc.

U.S. Cities and Their Nicknames

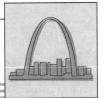

Not only do people have nicknames, but cities do also! Below are some of the nicknames of cities in the United States. Match them with the famous city on the right. Do you know any additional nicknames for the cities listed?

___ 1. The Gateway to the West

___ 2. America's Most Historic City

___ 3. The Windy City

___ 4. The Big Easy

___ 5. The Valley of the Sun

___ 6. The Mile High City

___ 7. The Big Apple

___ 8. The Emerald City

___ 9. The City of Brotherly Love

___ 10. Tinseltown

___ 11. Beantown

___ 12. The City of Angels

___ 13. The City of Roses

___ 14. Motown

___ 15. Sin City

___ 16. The Biggest Little City in the World

___ 17. The Twin Cities

___ 18. The City by the Bay

a. Phoenix

b. Hollywood

c. Los Angeles

d. Charleston

e. Denver

f. Chicago

g. San Francisco

h. New Orleans

i. Boston

j. Detroit

k. Minneapolis/St. Paul

l. St. Louis

m. Las Vegas

n. Reno

o. New York City

p. Philadelphia

q. Portland

r. Seattle

U.S. Cities and Their Nicknames ANSWER SHEET

1.	The Gateway to the West	l.	St. Louis
2.	America's Most Historic City	d.	Charleston
3.	The Windy City	f.	Chicago
4.	The Big Easy	h.	New Orleans
5.	The Valley of the Sun	a.	Phoenix
6.	The Mile High City	e.	Denver
7.	The Big Apple	o.	New York City
8.	The Emerald City	r.	Seattle
9.	The City of Brotherly Love	p.	Philadelphia
10.	Tinseltown	b.	Hollywood
11.	Beantown	i.	Boston
12.	The City of Angels	c.	Los Angeles
13.	The City of Roses	q.	Portland
14.	Motown	j.	Detroit
15.	Sin City	m.	Las Vegas
16.	The Biggest Little City in the World	n.	Reno
17.	The Twin Cities	k.	Minneapolis/St. Paul
18.	The City by the Bay	g.	San Francisco

FACILITATOR: *Many of the cities listed above are popular travel destinations. Ask participants if they have ever traveled to or lived in any of these cities. How do they think the cities got their nicknames (e.g., history, weather patterns, landmarks)? Do participants know the nicknames of any cities outside of the United States? For further discussion, have participants share the nicknames of the cities where they were born.*

Vacation Destinations

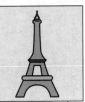

Most Americans love to travel, whether they are going to Grandmother's house 20 miles away or to the Far East. Travel magazines, books, and advertisements on the radio, on television, in magazines, and on the Internet all attempt to lure us to vacation destinations, both far and near. Identify the featured destinations based on the following descriptions.

1. What large stone wall stretches more than 4,000 miles and was largely built during the Ming Dynasty?

2. Which tower is approximately 984 feet tall, was completed in 1889, and is a great symbol of Paris?

3. What is the nickname of the large clock tower in London that is part of the Houses of Parliament?

4. An electronic ball drops from the top of a building in which famous square on New Year's Eve?

5. Which group of buildings in Moscow serves as the center of government?

6. What is the name of the location where the Pilgrims supposedly landed in 1620?

7. Which group of Washington, D.C., museums and galleries includes the National Air and Space Museum and the National Portrait Gallery?

8. Which 17th-century masterpiece is located in Agra, India, and was originally built as a mausoleum?

9. Which medieval building in Italy is famous for not being straight?

10. What wonder of the ancient world is located in Giza but is one of many such structures located throughout Egypt? (*Bonus:* What huge sculpture is located in front of the structure?)

11. Which Italian city is best known for its many canals and for its glass?

12. Which building, located on top of the Acropolis in Athens, Greece, was erected more than 2,000 years ago to honor Athena, the city's patron goddess?

13. What circle of mysterious stone structures is located in southern England?

14. Roman emperors built what famous amphitheater, which was host to gladiator fights, among other events?

15. Which Chinese city is home to an imperial palace referred to as the Forbidden City because entrance by commoners was once strictly prohibited?

16. Which city in Saudi Arabia is Islam's most holy city and is visited on a regular basis by Muslims from throughout the world?

Vacation Destinations ANSWER SHEET

1. What large stone wall stretches more than 4,000 miles and was largely built during the Ming Dynasty?
Great Wall of China

2. Which tower is approximately 984 feet tall, was completed in 1889, and is a great symbol of Paris?
Eiffel Tower

3. What is the nickname of the large clock tower in London that is part of the Houses of Parliament?
Big Ben

4. An electronic ball drops from the top of a building in which famous square on New Year's Eve?
Times Square

5. Which group of buildings in Moscow serve as the center of government?
Kremlin

6. What is the name of the location where the Pilgrims supposedly landed in 1620?
Plymouth Rock

7. Which group of Washington, D.C., museums and galleries includes the National Air and Space Museum and the National Portrait Gallery?
Smithsonian Institution

8. Which 17th-century masterpiece is located in Agra, India, and was originally built as a mausoleum?
Taj Mahal

9. Which medieval building in Italy is famous for not being straight?
Leaning Tower of Pisa

10. What wonder of the ancient world is located in Giza but is one of many such structures located throughout Egypt? (*Bonus:* What huge sculpture is located in front of the structure?)
Great Pyramid of Khufu (Sphinx)

11. Which Italian city is best known for its many canals and for its glass?
Venice

12. Which building, located on top of the Acropolis in Athens, Greece, was erected more than 2,000 years ago to honor Athena, the city's patron goddess?
Parthenon

13. What circle of mysterious stone structures is located in southern England?
Stonehenge

14. Roman emperors built what famous amphitheater, which was host to gladiator fights, among other events?
Coliseum

15. Which Chinese city is home to an imperial palace referred to as the Forbidden City because entrance by commoners was once strictly prohibited?
Beijing

16. Which city in Saudi Arabia is Islam's most holy city and is visited on a regular basis by Muslims from throughout the world?
Mecca

FACILITATOR: *The possibility for history lessons abounds with these tourist destinations! Using a map, locate each site. What is each place's history? Which participants have been to these locations? Create a list of what participants believe to be the 10 most popular tourist attractions in the world. If this activity is being used at a facility and there is room, try posting a world map and putting flags on all of the locations that participants have visited. Where would participants like to visit?*

Strengthen Your Mind by Einberger & Sellick. © 2007 by Health Professions Press, Inc.

Vegetables and Fruits

A world of tastes awaits you with these delicious descriptions. The foods described come from every corner of the earth, and eating them is a healthy way to keep your body and mind in good shape. While you are working on this sheet, think of the foods that are your old favorites as well as new ones that you may like to try.

1. Which tropical fruit, which grows on trees, will really hurt your head if it falls on you?

2. Which popular snack consists of peanut butter and raisins on top of a celery stick? (*Hint:* You probably had it as a child.)

3. One of which fruit per day will keep the doctor away?

4. Which sweet fruit is high in Vitamin C and is also a popular breakfast drink?

5. Sometimes mistaken for a vegetable, which red fruit may be sliced in a salad or topped with mozzarella and basil?

6. Which red, seeded fruit has a tough skin and is sometimes called "nature's most labor-intensive fruit"?

7. Native to tropical America, which fruit is black and tough on the outside and green and soft on the inside?

8. Which leafy vegetable, a favorite of Popeye, is high in iron and packed with vitamins?

9. Many people prefer to eat what kind of vegetables and fruits, which are grown without chemical pesticides or fertilizers?

10. Which starchy root vegetable is the second most consumed food in the United States and can be eaten baked, fried, stuffed, or mashed?

11. The leaves of which vegetable are delicious dipped in butter or mayonnaise? *Hint:* Keep eating down to the fleshy heart for the real treat!

12. The presence of what differentiates a fruit from a vegetable?

13. Many fruits and vegetables taste best without their skin; however, there are quite a few that you can eat with the skin on. List at least five.

14. Which tart, red fruit might you find on top of a hot fudge sundae or in a delicious pie?

Vegetables and Fruits ANSWER SHEET

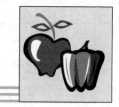

1. Which tropical fruit, which grows on trees, will really hurt your head if it falls on you?
   Coconut

2. Which popular snack consists of peanut butter and raisins on top of a celery stick? (*Hint:* You probably had it as a child.)
   Ants on a log

3. One of which fruit per day will keep the doctor away?
   Apple

4. Which sweet fruit is high in Vitamin C and is also a popular breakfast drink?
   Orange

5. Sometimes mistaken for a vegetable, which red fruit may be sliced in a salad or topped with mozzarella and basil?
   Tomato

6. Which red, seeded fruit has a tough skin and is sometimes called "nature's most labor-intensive fruit"?
   Pomegranate

7. Native to tropical America, which fruit is black and tough on the outside and green and soft on the inside?
   Avocado

8. Which leafy vegetable, a favorite of Popeye, is high in iron and packed with vitamins?
   Spinach

9. Many people prefer to eat what kind of vegetables and fruits, which are grown without chemical pesticides or fertilizers?
   Organic

10. Which starchy root vegetable is the second most consumed food in the United States and can be eaten baked, fried, stuffed, or mashed?
    Potato

11. The leaves of which vegetable are delicious dipped in butter or mayonnaise? *Hint:* Keep eating down to the fleshy heart for the real treat!
    Artichoke

12. The presence of what differentiates a fruit from a vegetable?
    Seeds

13. Many fruits and vegetables taste best without their skin; however, there are quite a few that you can eat with the skin on. List at least five.
    Apple, berries, carrot, cherry, cucumber, grape, nectarine, peach, pear, plum, potato, radish, tomato, yam

14. Which tart, red fruit might you find on top of a hot fudge sundae or in a delicious pie?
    Cherry

FACILITATOR: *For further discussion, make an A-to-Z list of fruits and one for vegetables. List fruits by season (e.g., summer fruits, winter fruits), and encourage participants to name their favorite fruits. You can also brainstorm the following lists: root vegetables, vegetables that are frequently mistaken for fruits, and fruits and vegetables by color.*

Strengthen Your Mind by Einberger & Sellick. © 2007 by Health Professions Press, Inc.

The Wild West

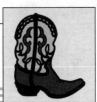

The days of the Wild West included cowboys, outlaws, stagecoaches, gun battles, ghost towns, and much more. Today, the West continues to intrigue people. Use your knowledge of this colorful period in history to answer the following questions.

1. Who was an expert rifle and shotgun markswoman of the Wild West?

2. Who was called the "King of the Wild Frontier"?

3. Name of the ranch where Bonanza takes place.

4. Which star of many westerns was nicknamed "The Duke"?

5. What is a Dead Man's Hand in poker?

6. Who was the Native American woman who helped guide Lewis and Clark?

7. What was the nickname of William Bonney, the infamous outlaw?

8. Who was known as "The Singing Cowboy"?

9. Which outfit provided mail delivery between Missouri and California?

10. What is the name of leather pants without a seat that are worn over other pants?

11. What is the location where many men died struggling for Texas's independence from Mexico?

12. Which popular vacation option is modeled after an authentic Western ranch?

13. Who conceived of the idea for the Wild West Show?

14. Which wagon held the cook and all of the food for a wagon train?

15. Doc Holliday and Wyatt Earp both took part in which famous fight?

16. Who was the Lone Ranger's faithful Native American companion?

17. Whose theme song was "Happy Trails to You"?

The Wild West ANSWER SHEET

1. Who was an expert rifle and shotgun markswoman of the Wild West?
    Annie Oakley

2. Who was called the "King of the Wild Frontier"?
    Davy Crockett

3. Name of the ranch where Bonanza takes place.
    Ponderosa

4. Which star of many westerns was nicknamed "The Duke"?
    John Wayne

5. What is a Dead Man's Hand in poker?
    Two aces and two 8s

6. Who was the Native American woman who helped guide Lewis and Clark?
    Sacagawea

7. What was the nickname of William Bonney, the infamous outlaw?
    Billy the Kid

8. Who was known as "The Singing Cowboy"?
    Gene Autry

9. Which outfit provided mail delivery between Missouri and California?
    Pony Express

10. What is the name of leather pants without a seat that are worn over other pants?
    Chaps

11. What is the name of the location where many men died struggling for Texas's independence from Mexico?
    Alamo

12. Which popular vacation option is modeled after an authentic Western ranch?
    Dude ranch

13. Who conceived of the idea for the Wild West Show?
    William "Buffalo Bill" Cody

14. Which wagon held the cook and all of the food for a wagon train?
    Chuckwagon

15. Doc Holliday and Wyatt Earp both took part in which famous fight?
    Gunfight at the OK Corral

16. Who was the Lone Ranger's faithful Native American companion?
    Tonto

17. Whose theme song was "Happy Trails to You"?
    Roy Rogers and Dale Evans

FACILITATOR: *The history of the Wild West is sure to bring up many memories of movies, television shows, books, and more. Great discussions may center around "good" guys versus "bad" guys, the role of women in the Wild West, gambling, favorite Western stars, and movies and television shows. Ask participants what it would have been like to live in this time and how it would have been different from today. Would participants have liked to live back then?*

Strengthen Your Mind by Einberger & Sellick. © 2007 by Health Professions Press, Inc.

World Continents and Countries

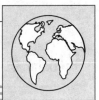

There are more than 190 countries in the world, located on seven continents. Most of us live in the third largest country in the world—the United States. Identify the following continents and countries.

1. What is the largest continent?

2. Which country is home of the Pyramids of Giza?

3. Which continent contains the most countries (53)?

4. La Paz, Santiago, and Lima are three capitals on which continent?

5. Which European country is shaped like a boot?

6. A famous landmark divided which country from 1961 to 1989?

7. What is the most populated country in the world?

8. What is the largest country in the world geographically?

9. The biggest potato famine in history occurred in the mid-1800s in which country?

10. What is the smallest country in the world?

11. According to the World Tourism Organization, what is the most visited country in the world?

12. Which country is also a continent?

13. Geographically, what is the largest country in North America?

14. Which continent contains the world's longest river?

15. Name the seven continents.

16. Name five countries in Europe.

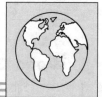

1. What is the largest continent?
   Asia (17,139,000 square miles)

2. Which country is home of the Pyramids of Giza?
   Egypt

3. Which continent contains the most countries (53)?
   Africa

4. La Paz, Santiago, and Lima are three capitals on which continent?
   South America

5. Which European country is shaped like a boot?
   Italy

6. A famous landmark divided which country from 1961 to 1989?
   Germany (Berlin Wall)

7. What is the most populated country in the world?
   China (more than 1,300,000,000 people)

8. What is the largest country in the world geographically?
   Russia

9. The biggest potato famine in history occurred in the mid-1800s in which country?
   Ireland

10. What is the smallest country in the world?
    Vatican City (0.2 square miles)

11. According to the World Tourism Organization, what is the most visited country in the world?
    France

12. Which country is also a continent?
    Australia

13. Geographically, what is the largest country in North America?
    Canada (3.9 million square miles)

14. Which continent contains the world's longest river?
    Africa (Nile River)

15. Name the seven continents.
    Africa, Asia, Antarctica, Australia, Europe, North America, South America

16. Name five countries in Europe.
    Check a map for answers.

FACILITATOR: *With a map, discussions about this topic can last for hours. Questions for participants include the following: Who has been to the most countries? Which countries would you like to visit? Which capitals can you name? How many countries can you name on each continent? What are some of these countries best known for? From which country or countries does your family originate?*

Xmas and Other Abbreviations

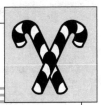

We use abbreviations to shorten a word (Dr. for *doctor)* or a group of words (USA for *United States of America).* Some of them are used in writing only while others are also used in speech. The following common abbreviations are used in everyday writing and speech. Identify the meaning of each abbreviation.

1.   Xmas

2.   AWOL

3.   IBM

4.   NAACP

5.   RN

6.   RSVP

7.   IQ

8.   CEO

9.   COD

10. NASA

11. NATO

12. ASAP

13. BA

14. GOP

15. IRS

16. lb.

17. mph

18. DOB

19. Ltd.

20. FBI

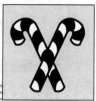

1.	Xmas	**Christmas**
2.	AWOL	**Absent without leave**
3.	IBM	**International Business Machines**
4.	NAACP	**National Association for the Advancement of Colored People**
5.	RN	**Registered nurse**
6.	RSVP	**Please reply (répondez s'il vous plaît, in French)**
7.	IQ	**Intelligence quotient**
8.	CEO	**Chief executive officer**
9.	COD	**Cash on delivery or Collect on delivery**
10.	NASA	**National Aeronautics and Space Administration**
11.	NATO	**North Atlantic Treaty Organization**
12.	ASAP	**As soon as possible**
13.	BA	**Bachelor of Arts**
14.	GOP	**Grand Old Party**
15.	IRS	**Internal Revenue Service**
16.	lb.	**Pound**
17.	mph	**Miles per hour**
18.	DOB	**Date of birth**
19.	Ltd.	**Limited**
20.	FBI	**Federal Bureau of Investigation**

FACILITATOR: The list of abbreviations is nearly endless. Ask participants for other examples. Additional questions include the following: What were some of the programs that Franklin Roosevelt developed that had abbreviations? Which abbreviations do you use most commonly? Do you ever make up your own abbreviations while writing notes? Do secretaries still use shorthand? Why or why not? Do you know any of the abbreviations associated with computers (e.g., www, @, PC, AOL)?

X-tremes of the World

From tall people, to high mountains, to fast cars, our world is full of extremes. The questions below deal with smaller- and larger-than-life people, animals, and events. Answer the following questions to explore the extremes of the world.

1. When it was completed in 1936, what 726-foot Arizona/Nevada dam was the highest in the United States?

2. Located at an elevation of 11,153 feet, what Colorado tunnel (named after a president) makes traveling across the continental divide easy?

3. Completed in 1965, what famous arch is 630-feet tall and welcomes visitors to the western half of the United States?

4. What gigantic shopping center located in Minnesota has more than 2.5 million square feet of retail space as well as an aquarium, wedding chapel, and theme park?

5. What tiny horses, which originated in Argentina, stand less than 30 inches tall but are sturdy and strong?

6. At 1,450 feet high, which Chicago building is the tallest in the United States?

7. At 282 feet below sea level, which California desert area is the lowest point in the United States?

8. Which animal is the fastest on land and can run for brief periods of time at speeds up to 70 mph?

9. On what continent was the lowest temperature, a frigid 128° below zero, recorded?

10. Which gigantic trees can reach heights of more than 270 feet with circumferences of more than 100 feet? (*Hint:* The largest is named General Sherman.)

11. Which theme park located in Orlando, Florida, is the largest in the world and covers an area of 30,000 acres?

12. Which tiny country is surrounded by Rome, Italy, and, at 0.2 square miles in size, is the smallest country in the world?

13. Standing at 20,320 feet high, which Alaskan mountain is the tallest in the United States?

14. What is the largest land mammal on earth? (*Hint:* It can grow up to 13 feet tall at the shoulder and weigh up to 12 tons.)

15. Which Hawaiian volcano is the world's largest and one of the most active? (*Hint:* It rises 13,680 feet above sea level and covers more than half of the island.)

X-tremes of the World ANSWER SHEET

1. When it was completed in 1936, what 726-foot Arizona/Nevada dam was the highest in the United States?
   Hoover Dam

2. Located at an elevation of 11,153 feet, what Colorado tunnel (named after a president) makes traveling across the continental divide easy?
   Eisenhower Tunnel

3. Completed in 1965, what famous arch is 630 feet tall and welcomes visitors to the western half of the United States?
   Gateway Arch (St. Louis, Missouri)

4. What gigantic shopping center located in Minnesota has more than 2.5 million square feet of retail space as well as an aquarium, wedding chapel, and theme park?
   Mall of America

5. What tiny horses, which originated in Argentina, stand less than 30 inches tall but are sturdy and strong?
   Falabella Horses

6. At 1,450 feet high, which Chicago building is the tallest in the United States?
   Sears Tower

7. At 282 feet below sea level, which California desert area is the lowest point in the United States?
   Death Valley

8. Which animal is the fastest on land and can run for brief periods of time at speeds up to 70 mph?
   Cheetah

9. On what continent was the lowest temperature, a frigid 128° below zero, recorded?
   Antarctica

10. Which gigantic trees can reach heights of more than 270 feet with circumferences of more than 100 feet? (*Hint:* The largest is named General Sherman.)
    Giant Sequoias

11. Which theme park located in Orlando, Florida, is the largest in the world and covers an area of 30,000 acres?
    Disney World

12. Which tiny country is surrounded by Rome, Italy, and, at 0.2 square miles in size, is the smallest country in the world?
    Vatican City

13. Standing at 20,320 feet high, which Alaskan mountain is the tallest in the United States?
    Mt. McKinley

14. What is the largest land mammal on earth? (*Hint:* It can grow up to 13 feet tall at the shoulder and weigh up to 12 tons.)
    Elephant (male African bush elephant)

15. Which Hawaiian volcano is the world's largest and one of the most active? (*Hint:* It rises 13,680 feet above sea level and covers more than half of the island.)
    Mauna Loa

FACILITATOR: *You might want to have a copy of the Guinness World Records on hand to look up other extremes while discussing this worksheet. Ask participants if anyone has ever attempted something extreme. If they could be in the Guinness World Records for any accomplishment, what would it be?*

Strengthen Your Mind by Einberger & Sellick. © 2007 by Health Professions Press, Inc.

Yo-Yos and Other Childhood Toys

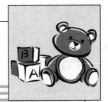

Though many toys have their beginnings in ancient history, like the yo-yo, the modern versions of the following toys were created in the late 19th century and throughout the 20th century. These toys are classics and continue to be popular today, for children, adults, and collectors. Match the toy on the right with the year it was invented and a description.

____ 1. 1902—This furry animal was named after the president at the time.

____ 2. 1903—This toy originally cost a nickel for a pack of eight.

____ 3. 1906—This motorized toy bears its inventor's middle name.

____ 4. 1913—This metal construction toy has evenly spaced holes for hardware to pass through.

____ 5. 1914—With these brightly colored wooden parts, children can build large structures, such as Ferris wheels, that actually move.

____ 6. 1916—These interlocking brown wooden pieces were created by John Lloyd Wright, son of architect Frank Lloyd Wright.

____ 7. 1919—Jumping was made easy by using this toy with springs.

____ 8. Early 1930s—This metal toy, which is ALWAYS red, had a wooden predecessor called the Liberty Coaster.

____ 9. 1939—This toy requires the additional purchase of reels.

____ 10. 1945—This steel toy can walk down stairs.

____ 11. 1947—This steel vehicle is built to last!

____ 12. 1948—This plastic disc cashed in on the growing popularity of UFOs.

____ 13. 1956—In the beginning, this toy was only produced in off-white, but in 1957 a three pack of red, blue, and yellow was offered.

____ 14. 1958—More than 20 million of these round, tubular toys were sold in the first 6 months of production.

____ 15. 1959—Named after the inventor's daughter, this toy has had dozens of makeovers since its inception.

a. Erector set

b. Tinkertoys

c. Frisbee

d. Crayola crayons

e. Tonka truck

f. Teddy bear

g. Lincoln Logs

h. Hula Hoop

i. Play-Doh

j. Slinky

k. View-Master

l. Radio Flyer

m. Barbie doll

n. Lionel train

o. Pogo stick

Yo-Yos and Other Childhood Toys ANSWER SHEET

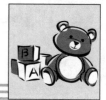

1. 1902—This furry animal was named after the president at the time.

    f.   **Teddy bear**

2. 1903—This toy originally cost a nickel for a pack of eight.

    d.   **Crayola crayons**

3. 1906—This motorized toy bears its inventor's middle name.

    n.   **Lionel train**

4. 1913—This metal construction toy has evenly spaced holes for hardware to pass through.

    a.   **Erector set**

5. 1914—With these brightly colored wooden parts, children can build large structures, such as Ferris wheels, that actually move.

    b.   **Tinkertoys**

6. 1916—These interlocking brown wooden pieces were created by John Lloyd Wright, son of architect Frank Lloyd Wright.

    g.   **Lincoln Logs**

7. 1919—Jumping was made easy by using this toy with springs.

    o.   **Pogo stick**

8. Early 1930s—This metal toy, which is ALWAYS red, had a wooden predecessor called the Liberty Coaster.

    l.   **Radio Flyer**

9. 1939—This toy requires the additional purchase of reels.

    k.   **View-Master**

10. 1945—This steel toy can walk down stairs.

    j.   **Slinky**

11. 1947—This steel vehicle is built to last!

    e.   **Tonka truck**

12. 1948—This plastic disc cashed in on the growing popularity of UFOs.

    c.   **Frisbee**

13. 1956—In the beginning, this toy was only produced in off-white, but in 1957 a three pack of red, blue, and yellow was offered.

    i.   **Play-Doh**

14. 1958—More than 20 million of these round, tubular toys were sold in the first 6 months of production.

    h.   **Hula Hoop**

15. 1959—Named after the inventor's daughter, this toy has had dozens of makeovers since its inception.

    m.   **Barbie doll**

FACILITATOR: This activity is sure to bring up many good memories of childhood. As you review each entry, ask participants the following questions: Did you have this toy? What do you remember about the toy? How much did it cost? What color was it? Who gave it to you? How popular was the toy? Is the toy still played with by children today? Ask participants for suggestions of other classic toys. These might include rocking horses, tops, building blocks, different types of dolls, and dollhouses. An extension to this activity is to ask participants to bring in toys that they still have from their childhood or pictures of such toys.

     Strengthen Your Mind by Einberger & Sellick. © 2007 by Health Professions Press, Inc.

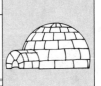

Yurts, Igloos, and Other Types of Shelters

A yurt is a portable, circular, domed shelter. Yurts were first used to house nomadic people in central Asia but are now being used as an alternative to other types of houses elsewhere. Identify the shelters described below.

1. What circular house is made of blocks of hard snow?

2. What residence on top of a tall building is usually inhabited by the wealthy?

3. What is a small, cozy house in the country called?

4. What portable structure is cone shaped and made from animal skins?

5. What is a small one-roomed apartment called?

6. Abraham Lincoln was born in what type of house, which is made from tree trunks?

7. A house divided into two separate residences is called what?

8. What type of residence is kept on the water, such as on a river?

9. A large, official house, often inhabited by a queen or king, is called what?

10. What type of roof, often found on English cottages, is made from straw or other vegetation?

11. A large residence built in the past to protect people inside from attack is called what?

12. What very large, expensive house is associated with wealthy people?

13. Multiple homes of similar design built next to one another are called what type of housing?

14. What type of house with a front of reddish brown stone is very common in New York?

15. What type of home is designed to be lived in while traveling?

16. What hollow or natural passage in the side of a mountain served as a dwelling for primitive man?

17. What type of house is a popular playhouse for children and also was home to the Swiss family Robinson?

18. In the children's story *The Three Little Pigs*, what three items did the pigs use to build their houses?

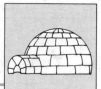

1. What circular house is made of blocks of hard snow?
    Igloo

2. What residence on top of a tall building is usually inhabited by the wealthy?
    Penthouse

3. What is a small, cozy house in the country called?
    Cottage

4. What portable structure is cone shaped and made from animal skins?
    Teepee

5. What is a small one-roomed apartment called?
    Studio or efficiency

6. Abraham Lincoln was born in what type of house, which is made from tree trunks?
    Log cabin

7. A house divided into two separate residences is called what?
    Duplex

8. What type of residence is kept on the water, such as on a river?
    Houseboat

9. A large, official house, often inhabited by a queen or king, is called what?
    Palace

10. What type of roof, often found on English cottages, is made from straw or other vegetation?
    Thatched roof

11. A large residence built in the past to protect people inside from attack is called what?
    Castle

12. What very large, expensive house is associated with wealthy people?
    Mansion

13. Multiple homes of similar design built next to one another are called what type of housing?
    Tract

14. What type of house with a front of reddish brown stone is very common in New York?
    Brownstone

15. What type of home is designed to be lived in while traveling?
    Motor home

16. What hollow or natural passage in the side of a mountain served as a dwelling for primitive man?
    Cave

17. What type of house is a popular playhouse for children and also was home to the Swiss family Robinson?
    Treehouse

18. In the children's story *The Three Little Pigs*, what three items did the pigs use to build their houses?
    Straw, sticks, and bricks

FACILITATOR: *This activity will most likely bring up discussions about different cultures and how people of these cultures live as well as thoughts and memories of participants' homes throughout their lifetimes. Ask participants to describe their first home. How big was it? How much did it cost? What was the yard like? Then, ask participants to describe their ideal home. What would it be like? Where would it be? Discuss how homes have changed over the years.*

Zip-A-Dee-Doo-Dah
and Other Lines from Famous Songs

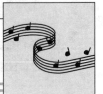

As they say, music is the universal language. It can bring us all together. It can change our mood. It can certainly help with our memory. The following lines are all lyrics from famous songs. Can you name the songs?

1. Where the deer and the antelope play

2. Where the treetops glisten and children listen

3. A real live nephew of my uncle Sam's

4. For amber waves of grain

5. Keep the love-light glowing in your eyes so true

6. I can't afford a carriage

7. If they don't win, it's a shame.

8. You're the emblem of the land I love.

9. With my banjo on my knee

10. Strolling through a shady lane

11. Tell all the gang at Forty-Second Street

12. In the lilt of Irish laughter

13. Snow time ain't no time to stay outdoors and spoon

14. From California to the New York Island

15. Through the night with a light from above

16. Chicks and ducks and geese better scurry

17. Another day older and deeper in debt

18. I'm going home to my city by the bay

Zip-A-Dee-Doo-Dah
and Other Lines from Famous Songs ANSWER SHEET

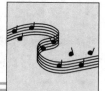

1. Where the deer and the antelope play
   Home on the Range

2. Where the treetops glisten and children listen
   White Christmas

3. A real live nephew of my uncle Sam's
   I'm a Yankee Doodle Dandy

4. For amber waves of grain
   America, the Beautiful

5. Keep the love-light glowing in your eyes so true
   Let Me Call You Sweetheart

6. I can't afford a carriage
   Bicycle Built for Two

7. If they don't win, it's a shame.
   Take Me Out to the Ball Game

8. You're the emblem of the land I love.
   (You're a) Grand Old Flag

9. With my banjo on my knee
   Oh! Susanna

10. Strolling through a shady lane
    In the Good Old Summertime

11. Tell all the gang at Forty-Second Street
    Give My Regards to Broadway

12. In the lilt of Irish laughter
    When Irish Eyes are Smiling

13. Snow time ain't no time to stay outdoors and spoon
    Shine on Harvest Moon

14. From California to the New York Island
    This Land Is Your Land

15. Through the night with a light from above
    God Bless America

16. Chicks and ducks and geese better scurry
    Surrey with the Fringe on Top

17. Another day older and deeper in debt
    Sixteen Tons

18. I'm going home to my city by the bay
    I Left My Heart in San Francisco

FACILITATOR: *Music is indeed the universal language. After participants answer these questions—or as they answer them if you do this activity as a group—you may want to sing each song together. Otherwise, ask for the rest of the lyrics. Who made each song famous? When was each song most popular? Ask participants about their favorite types of music, favorite songs, and favorite musicians.*

Strengthen Your Mind by Einberger & Sellick. © 2007 by Health Professions Press, Inc.

Zoos and Zoo Animals

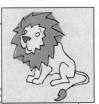

Zoos have been around for hundreds of years but have come a long way in the care and habitat of the animals. These days, many zoos have specialized landscapes that recreate an animal's natural environment and scientific programs to promote animal research. Answer the questions below to test your knowledge of various zoos and the animals that live in them.

1. What endangered species were Ling-Ling and Hsing-Hsing, who were given to the United States as a breeding pair but had no surviving offspring?

2. Which famous zoo in southern California is known for its tram ride and walking trails that let visitors see wild animals up close?

3. Which type of zoo is popular with children because it lets visitors touch and sometimes even feed the animals?

4. Which classification of animal can live on land and in the water but needs the warmth of the sun to be active?

5. Which type of zoo exhibits aquatic animals and plants, often for research and breeding purposes? (*Hint:* One of the most famous is located in Monterey Bay, California.)

6. Which popular zoo animal is the largest mammal on the planet? (*Hint:* It has a long trunk and enjoys bathing and playing in water.)

7. Which zoo is located in New York, has more than 4,000 animals on over 265 acres, and is known for its Wild Asia Tramway and Jungleworld?

8. *Shamu* is the icon of which marine park that has locations in Orlando, Florida; San Diego, California; and San Antonio, Texas?

9. Many animals like to live and travel in groups. What is a group of fish called?

10. What is a group of lions called?

11. What is a group of monkeys called?

12. What is a group of seals called?

13. What classification of animal, with more than 8,800 species, has hollow bones and feathers?

14. Which water-loving animal, found in the southeastern United States, can weigh up to 1,000 pounds and has a broad snout and powerful jaws?

15. What type of biology deals with animals?

16. The character Winnie the Pooh was based on what type of animal that lived at the London Zoo?

17. Which city is home to the first zoo in the United States?

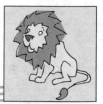

1. What endangered species were Ling-Ling and Hsing-Hsing, who were given to the United States as a breeding pair but had no surviving offspring?
   Giant pandas

2. Which famous zoo in southern California is known for its tram ride and walking trails that let visitors see wild animals up close?
   San Diego Zoo's Wild Animal Park

3. Which type of zoo is popular with children because it lets visitors touch and sometimes even feed the animals?
   Petting zoo

4. Which classification of animal can live on land and in the water but needs the warmth of the sun to be active?
   Amphibian

5. Which type of zoo exhibits aquatic animals and plants, often for research and breeding purposes? (*Hint:* One of the most famous is located in Monterey Bay, California.)
   Aquarium

6. Which popular zoo animal is the largest mammal on the planet? (*Hint:* It has a long trunk and enjoys bathing and playing in water.)
   Elephant

7. Which zoo is located in New York, has more than 4,000 animals on over 265 acres, and is known for its Wild Asia Tramway and Jungleworld?
   The Bronx Zoo

8. Shamu is the icon of which marine park that has locations in Orlando, Florida; San Diego, California; and San Antonio, Texas?
   Sea World

9. Many animals like to live and travel in groups. What is a group of fish called?
   School

10. What is a group of lions called?
    Pride

11. What is a group of monkeys called?
    Troop or barrel

12. What is a group of seals called?
    Pod

13. What classification of animal, with more than 8,800 species, has hollow bones and feathers?
    Bird

14. Which water-loving animal, found in the southeastern United States, can weigh up to 1,000 pounds and has a broad snout and powerful jaws?
    Alligator

15. What type of biology deals with animals?
    Zoology

16. The character Winnie the Pooh was based on what type of animal that lived at the London Zoo?
    Black bear

17. Which city is home to the first zoo in the United States?
    Philadelphia

FACILITATOR: *Encourage participants to talk about their experiences at zoos. Which zoos have they visited? Do they have favorite animals? Do they agree with the idea of zoos? Make an A-to-Z list of animals you would find at a zoo, and discuss endangered animals.*

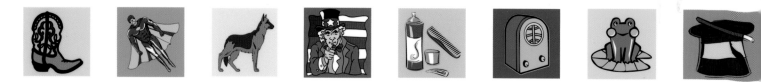

Strengthen Your Mind with more than 70 engaging activities! This collection of short, one-page worksheets will enhance brain functioning and sharpen memory skills. You'll have fun completing the activities by yourself or with a group of people.

Featuring trivia, reminiscence, and sensory stimulation, the activities engage multiple parts of the brain. You'll test your memory and gain new knowledge with matching, fill-in-the-blank, and brainstorming worksheets. And for questions that prove too much of a challenge, answer keys are provided.

Have fun remembering or discovering
- popular culture of former decades
- famous movie quotes
- historical people and places
- familiar advertising slogans
- favorite foods and beverages
- beloved fictional characters
- prominent world and U.S. landmarks
- and much more

These fun-filled activities will provide hours of enjoyment and valuable exercise for your brain.

Strengthen Your Mind is also a valuable resource for activity staff in senior centers, adult day services, and long-term care facilities. All activities have been field tested with individuals with early memory loss and include tips to promote engagement and group interaction.

"Accolades to Kristin Einberger and Janelle Sellick for researching and penning this wonderful exploration of remaining memories . . . Every family should have a copy of *Strengthen Your Mind* and all community-based programs (assisted living, adult day health, long-term care and others) should use this marvelous tome in daily programming."
—Joanne Koenig Coste,
author, *Learning to Speak Alzheimer's*

"Offering a treasure trove of interesting, informative, and enjoyable material, the book builds upon the growing emphasis in the dementia care field to recognize the capabilities of people with memory loss, and find ways to enhance them."
—Robyn Yale, L.C.S.W.,
Clinical Social Worker &
Early Stage Alzheimer's Consultant

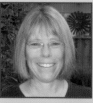
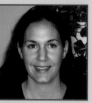

ABOUT THE AUTHORS:
Kristin Einberger and **Janelle Sellick, M.S.,** have more than 40 years of combined experience working with older adults with memory loss. They have developed educational/social programs for people with memory loss and their families and taught numerous memory enhancement classes.

ISBN 1-932529-31-4

9 781932 529319

90000

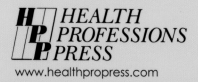

HEALTH PROFESSIONS PRESS

www.healthpropress.com